WHAT OTHERS ARE SAYING ABOUT MICHELLE THIELEN, YOGAFAITH, AND *STRETCHING YOUR FAITH*

"This book is a blueprint for what the Bible repeatedly declares Christ followers to do: rest, be still, meditate and worship with the whole mind, body, spirit and soul. Michelle has brilliantly weaved movement and scriptures into an eloquent flow of grace. Practicing what you read throughout these pages will leave you transformed from the inside and out."

Patrick Snow
Publishing Coach and International Best-Selling Author of *Creating Your Own Destiny*

"*Stretching Your Faith* is a perfect book to use as a companion for any teacher training program or to simply deepen one's own practice. Using powerful yoga poses, this book empowers you to take your health and well-being into your own hands, to gently ease your way into inner calm and happiness."

Susan Friedmann, CSP
International best-selling author of *Riches in Niches: How to Make it BIG in a small Market*

"Throughout these pages you will discover truths on how to silence the chaos that surrounds you on a daily basis. In reading this book you will experience a new found peace as you clear out the clutter and begin to move freely and breathe again. This amazing resource is a comprehensive guide that offers hundreds of postures with many variations shown so that anyone and everyone can enjoy yoga. It is also ideal for teacher training to take your mastery of yoga to a higher level."

Nicole Gabriel
Author of *Finding Your Inner Truth and Certified Yoga Instructor*

"Yoga and Jesus are two of my favorite things in the world! I am enlightened and forever changed by Michelle and her beautiful soul. Thank you for forever changing my life."

Renee Gillard
Author of *No More Insulin*

"*Stretching Your Faith* embodies a holistic approach to worship. You will create the most intimate space possible with the Lord by putting into practice worship with your entire body and strength. This Spirit led guide will change your life."

Frank Reed
Author of *In God We Trust Dollars and Sense*. Speaker and Coach, Bottomline Ministries

"Michelle seamlessly blends her passion for Jesus with her passion for yoga. Her classes are worshipful and welcoming for yogis of any faith journey. The YogaFaith practice has blessed many in our community."

Gae Dougherty,
Senior Director of Health and Well Being, Mel Korum YMCA, WA

"As an author of expanding joy, *Stretching Your Faith* will align any 'body' into a physical discipline, but more than that, these pages will help you achieve lasting change in every area of your life."

Brett Dupree
Author of *Joyous Expansion; Unleashing Your Passion to Lead an Inspired Life*

"Michelle is an amazing woman of God who has a passion for serving the less fortunate. In the years that I have known her, she radiates a positive, filled-with-the-spirit perspective on the world. Truly a light on a mountain top. Her dedication to showing God's love and mercy makes me feel honored to know her. The work that she provides in allowing one to focus on God, facilitating intimacy with our Creator, as well as getting our body 'whole', is what more people need in this world. There is nothing quite like YogaFaith, it is something you must experience, and you will throughout the pages of *Stretching Your Faith*."

Eli Struck
Founder of Enlighting Struck Design

"*Stretching Your Faith* demystifies Christians practicing yoga. These pages are filled with an in-depth richness of reclaiming and redeeming Biblical principles."

Sarah Quinton
Author of *Excelling in Service*

"*Stretching Your Faith* brought together my love of Jesus and my love of yoga. The direction of my life changed when I learned that I could continue my yoga practice in worship and praise. Previously I struggled with reconciling my faith and the practice of yoga, Michelle clearly lays out how you can redeem your yoga practice by putting Jesus first. In no ambiguous terms this book clearly puts Jesus and the word of God before the postures, while teaching you to use your whole body in worship, giving new meaning to the words "moving meditation." *Stretching Your Faith* has helped me to pray more wholly by giving me understanding of the postures of prayer. After reading this book I confidently practice yoga as a part of my spiritual growth and relationship with the Lord."

Leanne Winslow, RYT, R-YFT
YogaFaith Instructor

"*Stretching Your Faith* brings great synchronization between mind, body spirit, and soul. You will find yourself immersed spiritually as well as physically. Michelle is an amazing woman of God and yoga teacher. She has great passion to propel the Kingdom of God as she boldly lives out her God-inspired life. Whenever I take a YogaFaith class, I find myself immersed in HIS presence. The atmosphere is so angelic. Michelle has such a gentle calm spirit. You will leave inspired and renewed.
Thank you, Michelle, for launching YogaFaith as well as *Stretching Your Faith*. It's an amazing yoga practice that is all about connecting your whole-being with Christ."

Glenda McGowen Shepard, ARNP, MSA, CPT
Holistic Wellness Practitioner, Yoga Studio Owner, Triumphant Strength Ministries

"If you love Jesus and yoga, this is the only book you need to read. It is so thorough in biblical principles with a vast, in-depth knowledge of hundreds of postures and all of their modifications. I have explored postures throughout these pages that I never knew existed. In *Stretching Your Faith* every stone is turned and light is shined on ancient mysteries from yoga and the history of the Word of God."

Renee Kay
Author and Professional Speaker

"Michelle brings her deep rooted faith, charismatic and passionate spirit to the disciplines and traditions of yoga inviting all walks of faith to engage in a fully present practice in body, mind and spirit onto their yoga mat through a purposeful spiritual alignment on each page of this inspiring and comprehensive educational book. *Stretching Your Faith* demystifies any doctrinal misgivings and invites a new found freedom to worship without judgment in a language that allows believers to embrace their faith at a deeper level, explore and stretch their faith through body and mind techniques."

Gina Tricamo, E-RYT 500, MLC
Global Growth Life Coaching

"*Stretching Your Faith* is a refreshing approach to yoga training. I was looking for a program that would compliment my commitment to posture and alignment but would consider the mind and the spirit as equals. YogaFaith's book is a comprehensive guide to a mind, body, and spirit connection that honors a commitment to Christ. Michelle incorporates many yoga philosophies without compromising Christian beliefs. She honors the century old traditions of yoga with a 2000 year old Biblical worldview. Michelle has successfully integrated the mind, body, and spirit tradition of yoga fused with the beliefs of Christianity that invites the Holy Spirit into the center of it all."

DiAnne Bergmann, BA, MME, RYT, R-YFT

"I have been waiting for a practical guide to lead me into not only a Christian approach to yoga, but an authentic way to spend time in devotions with God. *Stretching Your Faith* is it. I finally found a way to create space and time for Christ as well as keep Him the center of a physical practice that encompasses the Holy Spirit so profoundly. This book is transformational in every way!"

John Christopher Bryant
Author of *Women and Wealth*

"As a Christian, *Stretching Your Faith* has made it possible to practice yoga in a very sacred space with the Lord. I feel as if this is the first time I've ever been so intimate with Christ!"

Elisa Hawkinson
Author of *Calming Your Chaos*

"When one experiences Michelle's leadership in a yoga class you soon realize that she is committed to the practice of yoga, and helping others to realize their potential. I have become more confident in my practice through her challenges and encouragement. There are many unique gifts that Michelle brings to those she instructs, but the most powerful is inspiring the worship of God through yoga. Michelle ushers in the presence of the Holy Spirit throughout class, in postures of stillness and active movement, it really does not get any better than this. Thank you Michelle, and God bless you."

Reverend, Dr. Condry Robbins, II, PHD

"YogaFaith makes me happy! This program presents a strong connection between us and our Creator. Michelle emphasizes God's desire to communicate with us and clearly outlines the role yoga plays in our worship and surrender to Him. Going through this program not only strengthens our bodies, but draws us into a closer relationship with the One who uniquely designed us for this purpose."

Mary Doelman, MA
Counseling and Therapist. Christian Apologetics

"I went to a YogaFaith class near Christmas 2013 and was moved by the Spirit in a powerful way that evening. When I entered the room, the only spot available was at the foot of the Cross. I know the God orchestrated that just for me! There in the sacred space, I found release, stillness, and peace. Tears flowed from the beauty of encountering the Lord. My faith was stretched, strengthened and secured. Thank you Michelle for being His hands, feet and very breath."

Theresa A. Devers
Dietitian, Certified Health Coach, TNT Wellness Consulting, LLC

"YogaFaith showed me how to step out of the chaos of life and into stillness on the mat with God. On the mat I find healing, connection and a strength that only He can provide."

Julie Englund
Counselor and YogaFaith Student

"Jesus has demonstrated His grace and acceptance of who I am through YogaFaith, where worship is a lifestyle and a culture. He has provided me with the freedom to worship Him in all rhythms of life. He has reminded me through YogaFaith that I do not have to perform to earn His love, I am free to rest in Him, to just be. I am reminded to surrender my body and heart in unison and to depend on His Spirit. It has been very therapeutic to allow God into deep places in my heart where He is bringing hope and healing. I have enjoyed the many sweet times in classes and nature, connecting with God, His creation, and friends. It has been so refreshing to be around other people who also adore Jesus with their whole hearts. I have received so much love and care that I hope to share with others what I have learned through YogaFaith to make more disciples of Jesus Christ."

Alyse Rogers, R-YFT, RYT,
Master of Arts, Mental Health Counselor Associate

"*Stretching Your Faith* praises God in the stillness of prayer and in the active joy of movement. To be present with God and His word upon my yoga mat is a powerful promise of my breath and my heart's willing to surrender to His Divine plan. I have experienced no better way to see one's self than in the resting space of God's glory. He always shows up! He is my intention! My God, my mat, my community & me is YogaFaith. The scholarship and dedication of founder Michelle Thielen is unprecedented. She invests in your success, your developing clarity of vision and the application of becoming a God-driven 'change the world' impact-your-students Yoga Teacher! Your heart, and yoga tool box will be overflowing with all you have to offer. You will be ready, and you will have mentors for life cheering, praying and supporting. Show up and prepare to have your world rocked! You are so worth this experience! The greatest calling of my life thus far and I intend to listen!"

Sarah Willett, RYT, R-YFT
YogaFaith Trainer

"YogaFaith was exactly what I was looking for in my search for a certified teacher training! It gave me the opportunity to become certified and recognized by the Yoga Alliance while using the Bible as my textbook! My heart's desire was to teach yoga in a way that students could worship and focus on their Creator in spirit, mind, and body while they practiced on their mat in the "sacred space." That's what *Stretching Your Faith* and YogaFaith is all about! I am so grateful for Michelle's listening heart!"

Celeste Davidson, R-YFT, RYT
YogaFaith Ambassador, Kelowna, Canada BC

"YogaFaith is bridging the gap for so many yogis. Many people have no idea that they could center their yoga practice on Christ. After going through Michelle's program, I have not only achieved the skills necessary in teaching YogaFaith, I am equally confident in teaching many different styles of yoga. I think the best part of *Stretching Your Faith* and YogaFaith is that students become teachers, you will leave the program with a genuine love of the practice and for your students."

Meghan Mulholland, R-YFT, RYT
YogaFaith Instructor

"Michelle is one of those people I look up to and respect deeply. She serves others with her whole heart. Her passion in life is to teach yoga, faith in God, and is a wonderful role model encouraging others to pursue their God-given purpose. I feel very blessed to work alongside Michelle!"

Krista Butler RN, BSN, RYT, ACE
Health Coach, YogaFaith Prenatal and Yin Teacher Trainer, Founder of Stretching for Two

"Yoga and praising God at the same time, incredibly amazing!"

Sue Stults
Author of *Reaching Beyond the Rail, The Blood Sweat and Tears Of Caring for Mom and Dad*

"I really, really enjoyed this training. My heart is changed and definitely my yoga is changed, all wonderfully new! I really am almost out of words of praise for this experience. How Michelle pulled this all together is commendable. So much research between the Bible and yoga teachings really gave me a solid base to move forward combining my faith with my classes. I don't think I could have done it without her. The desire was there, but I didn't know how to bring this out confidently. Now I do. And, to get my 200RYT also is a dream come true. I have tried for so many years to finish my trainings, but it never worked out. Now, I know that God wanted me to wait to find YogaFaith. It was perfect for me and I couldn't imagine taking my 200RYT at any other school."

Carrie Morash, R-YFT, RYT
YogaFaith Trainer

"YogaFaith's motto is Jesus first, yoga second and that is exactly what you will experience throughout these pages. Michelle infuses a crazy amount of learning Jesus and yoga into these masterful pages. There is never a doubt that Jesus is first in her life and this evident throughout *Stretching Your Faith*. This practice can be used as a curriculum as it is extremely thorough. There was never a question or a circumstance where I felt out of place, as I flow in His grace I realize that I am exactly where I need to be, and you will find this perfect peace too. Training with Michelle was in God's perfect timing for me and He hooked me up! Thank you Michelle for being true to your mission and to us, your new yogis."

Bo Wilkinson , R-YFT
Integrative Nutrition Coach and YogaFaith Instructor

"I highly recommend *Stretching Your Faith* without reservation. I cannot put into words what this practice will do for you personally, spiritually, and professionally."

Holly Neal, R-YFT, RYT
YogaFaith Trainer

"YogaFaith has been an incredible journey. When I met Michelle and learned of Jesus and yoga, in addition to helping traffick survivors, I knew immediately I wanted to be a part of this movement. *Stretching Your Faith* teaches the power of worshiping God physically, mentally, emotionally and spiritually through yoga. Since my YogaFaith Training, I have been supported and encouraged to share Christ centered yoga in numerous venues. It has been such an incredible journey and it continually reminds me that there is healing for all who are hurting. YogaFaith teaches me to be still, to worship God with every cell in me, to love passionately and that we are created so perfectly, complete and whole in Jesus' eyes."

Jessica Dahl, R-YFT
Hair Stylist and YogaFaith Trainer

"Thanks, Michelle! You are a gem, a blessing, and a life-changer! Thank you for stepping out and taking your leap of faith that others like me can be inspired to do the same. Thank you for pouring your life into your students. The YogaFaith teacher training is a life-changing experience. This is more than excellent yoga teacher training (which it is), it is life changing! The learning is comprehensive, helping the student to learn, grow, and stretch their faith in new ways. The trainers are deep, loving, and ultra encouraging. If you are wondering if this training might be for you, IT IS!"

Louise Stanton, R-YFT, RYT
YogaFaith Trainer

"I would highly recommend this for anyone that has a passion for Christ and Yoga. YogaFaith is one of the best experiences of my life! Wonderful teacher Michelle loves Christ, yoga and loves to serve others. "

Kim Mulholland, R-YFT, RYT
YogaFaith Trainer

"Using yoga as a spiritual practice, *Stretching Your Faith* helps clear the chaos and clutter and make space for movement in your life."

Gabriela Condrea
Author of *When 1+1=1*, Founder of Connection Through Movement

"I absolutely love my time with YogaFaith! It exceeded all my expectations and gave me the confidence to go out and teach others right away. Michelle is amazing and encouraging on so many levels. The information within these pages is life changing in the best way possible! It will cause you to be hopeful for the future and of course fall even more in love with Jesus, yoga and others. Thank you Michelle for encouraging all of us to stretch our faith!"

Kelly Calkins, R-YFT, RYT
YogaFaith Trainer

A Self-leadership and Spirit-led Blueprint
to Experiencing Lasting Transformation

STRETCHING YOUR FAI†H

Practicing Postures of Prayer to Create
Peace, Balance and Freedom

MICHELLE THIELEN

Founder of YogaFaith.org

Love the Lord your God with all your heart,
with all your soul,
with all your strength,
and with all your mind.
Luke 10:27 God's Word Translation

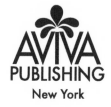

AVIVA
PUBLISHING
New York

STRETCHING YOUR FAITH

Practicing Postures of Prayer to Create Peace, Balance and Freedom

Published by:
Aviva Publishing
Lake Placid, NY
(518) 523-1320
www.AvivaPubs.com

ISBN: 978-1-48357-055-6

Library of Congress: 2015903942

Cover Designer: Eli Struck / Enlighting Struck Design, www.enlightingdesign.com

Cover Photo: Lucien Knuteson / Lucien Knuteson Photography, www.lucienknuteson.com

Interior Book Layout: Eli Struck / Enlighting Struck Design, www.enlightingdesign.com

Author Photo: Dee Jones, Open Door Photography, www.opendoorphotography.com

Every attempt has been made to properly source all quotes and bible translations.
Bible verses used are from the New International Version (NIV) Bible unless otherwise stated.

Printed in the Unites States of America
First Edition

DEDICATION

To the most amazing human I have ever known: my husband and best friend, Derek Thielen. God created you specifically for me. You are living proof that I did something right in my lifetime. I love you with my whole being; every fiber of me loves every fiber of you. One plus one equals one. Forever, one.

To my parents who gave me life. Dad, thank you for your love and support through the years. No matter what I choose to do, you cheer me on. Mom, I would not be alive without you. You breathed wind into my wings when life sucked it out of me. Your unconditional love, support, encouragement, and friendship have kept me going every day of my life. Because of your passion for the Lord, the light He has given you that shines brightly wherever you go, this living example of Him in you, showed me how to make Him the center of everything. How do I thank someone who not only gave me life, but also led me to the One who created life itself? I am forever grateful that God gave me you for this lifetime. All my heart and soul, Mishy Anna.

To you, the reader and my new friend. I dedicate this labor of love to you. I pray that with this practice of whole worship and complete surrender, you will experience intimacy with Christ like no other time in your life. I hope that in your times of stillness with Him, you will draw nearer to His heart and hear what He has to say to you in such a time as this. I pray that you hear His Spirit speak to yours as He beckons His children to rise up and ignite a revival throughout this generation. The plan of God requires that you hear from Him. I pray you're listening.

To Jesus Christ, my personal Lord and Savior. I dedicate these writings that Your very Spirit breathed through me to compose. I surrender these pages back to You, that Your will would be done with every word. More importantly, I dedicate my life to You as my gratitude for rescuing me from the pits of hell and the very clasp of the enemy's grip. He almost had me, but because You reached down, saved me, redeemed me, and turned everything around to work in my favor, I want every breath to glorify and honor You for the rest of my days. I want my life to point to You. Here I am, Lord; send me and keep sending me.

ACKNOWLEDGMENTS

Mary Hardy, Derek Thielen, John and Debbie Hardy, Jessica Dahl, Joyce Meyer, Joycelyn Hoober, Kelly Calkins, Marilyn Christianson, Melanie Hendershot, Krista Butler, Kristi Roy, Dee Jones, Leanne Winslow, David Wakeling, Steven Wong Jr. and Patrick Snow.

To the many students, instructors and mentors that have taught me, there are too many to list.
You have spoken to my heart and spirit influencing who I am today,
I acknowledge you and thank you for such immeasurable gifts.

Most importantly, my sincere gratitude to the Lord. I will spend the rest of my life singing Your praises for all that You have brought me through and where You are leading me now, it is a well watered land. Thank You for the wisdom to constantly stretch my faith.
To You all the glory, forever and ever.

CONTENTS

PREFACE

Our worlds can be so loud, noisy, hectic and completely overwhelming. We barely have time to sit down to pee, let alone find time to be still and alone with the Lord. This is exactly how the enemy would love to keep you, overwhelmed and frazzled with no room for distractions and interruptions, definitely no time for God and all that He has to communicate to you!

Have you ever had time to be still? You may laugh at the very word. "Still, what does that mean?" There is nothing the enemy would love more than for you to be so overwhelmed and busy that you cannot find time to be still or more importantly, be quiet enough to hear God's still small voice. After all, B.U.S.Y, you know stands for Buried Under satan's Yoke. When did you last read that God shouted anything? I cannot find anywhere in the word of God that He yelled when trying to speak to His people. The Lord and His spirit always speak gently, a whisper, usually in a "still small voice." The problem today is that we cannot hear Him. The single most dangerous thing to the god of this world, is that we hear from our God. As children of God the most important thing in our lives is to hear from the Lord. You must take time to be still and listen, it's too important not to. God will bless the rest of your day more abundantly when you seek Him first more than had you not spent the precious time with Him at all.

Are you able to hear God's still small voice among the chaos of today's loud world? Because you were created to hear from your Creator. Have you ever experienced such intimate and distraction-free worship? You were created for worship. When was the last time you completely surrendered your all and your will? Are you ready to deepen your walk with Christ, hear from Him and have hidden mysteries, treasures and wonders revealed to you? He is trying to communicate to His children. He has things He needs you to hear and know. You have places to go, things to do and people to meet! Maybe you are ready to encounter God for the very first time, or long for a fresh encounter with the Living Waters? Would you like to get healthy and whole once and for all? Are you willing to be transformed from the inside out? Awesome! I was hoping you would say yes!

I want to share how your life can be truly transformed by the Living Christ and the amazing gift of yoga. Do not be afraid of the word yoga, it simply means to be united, or to yoke. It is not our business how others use yoga or what they set their hearts and minds to while practicing yoga. Here, we set our hearts and minds on Jesus Christ and nobody should be able to judge how others worship. I believe God created everything in the Heavens and on the Earth. Therefore, I believe God created our body, how we move and physical activity that includes stretching our body. Release anything that is connected with the word yoga, except for what it truly means, to unite or yoke.

The combination of your faith, and literally stretching your faith, can heal your body, your mind, your spirit, marriage, relationships, business, ministry and so much more. You can be made whole by practicing the principles throughout these pages. Every area of your life can be healed, redeemed, restored and made new!

I began my yoga journey about 20 years ago as a means to prevent injury while professionally dancing. Throughout my dance career, yoga not only helped me to maintain my flexibility and strength with no injury, I soon discovered that it was a physical activity like no other.

When I attended yoga classes, often an instructor would incorporate a philosophy such as self enlightenment or tell students to honor "the source" within us. I would always think, "Yes the Source is within me, it is Christ alone, not me, but Him!" God always whispered to me to keep my heart and mind on Him. My yoga practice began to be Christ centered, but in a silent way. I longed to share what He was working in my heart, body and spirit with others. During an annual fast, God spoke to my heart to start YogaFaith. YogaFaith is a Christ centered approach to the practice of yoga. It is the ability to worship and surrender, fully and completely, perhaps in a way that you may have never worshiped before. It is also the practice of being still. It is the act of breathing the Holy Spirit into every fiber of our being as we breathe, as we move, exist and have our being (Acts 17:28). It is the opportunity to become united and yoked to Christ. When was the last time you were still long enough to hear from God? I can tell you that silence will bring you to His voice like nothing else.

My desire is what God has birthed deep down inside of me come to pass in my lifetime, that a nation and a generation begin taking time to seek God, hang out with Him, to hear from Him, to breathe His Spirit into their lives and atmospheres. That God would become the center of everyday, not just Sunday.

I am still on this journey with Him and though I do not have all the answers, the only important thing is that I know the One who holds all the answers. YogaFaith will become your prayers, set in motion so that you may flow in His grace. My hope for you is that YogaFaith draws you nearer to Him in this same way, I pray that you would then share and extend the gift of grace and 'prayers in motion' with others, ultimately taking Christ and the power of connecting to Him in whole worship and complete surrender, into a dark, lost and hurting world. Your loved ones need you to be whole, the world needs your gifts and God's plan requires that you hear from Him.

Are you ready for true transformation?

INTRODUCTION

Transformational Stretching

We are too busy. We are overwhelmed, exhausted and often times completely frazzled. The very things that God has blessed us with have become burdens and often times idols. It is time for us to get back to the basics. Together, let us lay aside all distractions, chaos and clutter. Instead let's create a space for peace, freedom, balance and rest. This book is much more than stretching your faith. It is an invitation into transformation. Should you accept the invitation, these pages will lead you into such an intimate space with Christ that you will leave changed from the inside out. You are about to enter a journey that offers whole worship and complete surrender like you have never experienced before.

You may be so out of balance that you often feel like life is spinning out of control. You crave sanity. You are not quite sure the last time you felt freedom. Do you feel like you are just going through the motions? Perhaps you are beyond autopilot with your job, family, church and other activities that you used to love. Do you resent the job that you once rejoiced over? Has it become a mundane routine or perhaps it is suffocating your God-given dreams? Sometimes we become so bored with going through the motions that we daydream of leaving it all behind, to start fresh in a new place, or we fantasize about moving to a cottage on the beach just for a little peace and quiet. You long to have just five minutes alone in complete silence. You have forgotten what peace feels like. Balance is a foreign word. Being still is impossible.

Like millions of people, you may suffer from discouragement, anxiety or a lack of peace. Perhaps, like many of us, you feed your discouragement with addictions such as food, shopping or alcohol. Do you have [any] margin in your day for when things don't go as they should? Or are you addicted to your "to do" list with no time for interruptions? Have you become so task oriented that your health and relationships have suffered or don't exist at all? Are you so frazzled that your loved ones have to walk on eggshells around you? Do you wander aimlessly because you have lost something, someone or maybe you have lost everything? Perhaps you're like me and lost everything more than once?

Somewhere along the pathway you lost 'you' and your joy. Perhaps you've reached the point where the once treasured gift of spending time with God has become a burden to you and maybe just flat out doesn't even sound good anymore. Besides, you have too much 'to do' to take time to hang out with God! I have good news for you, together we are going to reclaim our joy, our peace, balance, time and our freedom. We are going to redeem our mind, body, spirit and souls! You and I are going to separate from the cocoon, spread our beautiful wings and fly into the destiny that God has prepared for us.

We are all in the same boat. Life is busy and can be a constant struggle. The pressures of today's world to "do", gather, produce and achieve are overwhelming. We get discouraged if we are not successful as the world defines success. Life can be hopeless and depressing. This world can be a dark and lonely place. I have been to these dark and lonely places. I have been so far out on the ledge that giving up seemed to be the easiest way out. It seems so simple to stop trying and just let go. Trust me when I tell you, I understand. I know what it feels like to lose absolutely everything. In 2004 I was so depressed, discouraged and hopeless that taking my own life seemed the easiest route. The only reason I didn't is so that I could live to tell you that there is hope! There is a way up and a way out for you. His name is Jesus and He can take any mess and turn it into a message of hope and redemption. He promises to bring you out, give you hope and make a way! I am here to tell you that everything is going to be okay and I see a turnaround in your near future! It may not be easy climbing out of the pit, but it will be worth it! Your testimony will glorify God and give others hope. Each one of us have to go through a struggle in the difficult, dark and lonely cocoon for one reason, and that is to glorify God who brings us out of the darkness. Are you ready to go from the pit to the palace?

During our time together, you will learn how your life can be truly transformed. You will learn how to be still, how to hear from and be sensitive to the Holy Spirit. You will learn how to meditate on Christ, just as the Word declares, and why this is so vital as a Christian. You will experience hundreds of postures that will bring life and health to every cell and fiber of your body. You will develop life changing habits that will prolong your life span and create a healthy atmosphere for you, your family, your home and all your relationships. If you put into practice what we explore on these pages, your peace, joy, balance and freedom will be reclaimed. You will also learn several different breathing techniques and regain the ability to breathe again. Breathing the Holy Spirit into the innermost parts of your physical, spiritual, relational and emotional 'home'. You will also develop a God-confidence that only comes from spending time with the Lord. We become like those we hang out with and you will develop a joyous habit of hanging out with God, hearing from Him and all the things that He has for you, as well as shining your unique light into the world so that you too can help a dark and lost generation. He will bless the rest of the day beyond your wildest imagination if you sacrifice your first fruits with Him.

God has designed you uniquely. You contain special gifts and talents that nobody else has and my prayer is that you will use those gifts to glorify God and point others toward Him. Lastly, as we journey together, I want to invite you to resist the urge to "constantly accomplish." Why is it that at the end of a day if we are not completely exhausted we feel like a failure? I absolutely hate the word busy. When you ask someone how they are doing and their reply is "busy", it drives me crazy. We not only need to take this word out of our vocabulary, we need to be intentional about getting UN-busy! Let's encourage one another to resist the urge to always continue, produce and accomplish. To honor God's instruction of a Sabbath rest. We need rest. It's okay to unplug and disconnect. Yes, unplug, disconnect so that you may plug into the True Source. Create space and time for loved ones, service and devotion. That is why Sabbath exists: rest, devotion, service and worship.

There is a very real enemy that roams the earth seeking to devour. He wants our family, our dreams and our joy to be broken and shattered to smithereens. Life happens. I understand, hearts are broken, dreams get buried and the happily-never-happened goes to our graves with us if we don't do something about it. If you put your dreams on hold to raise a family, perhaps it's time to breathe life back into your dreams. Perhaps you have been mourning the passing of a loved one and it's time for you to start living again. I don't know what it is, but I'm here to tell you that because you are here, heart beating, air-in-the-lungs-still-here, you have something else to do! Now is the time, this is the place and you are the one! I believe in you. And if you are the only one that has to stir yourself up today, so be it! Start speaking life into the dead places. Choose life giving words over your days. Stop putting photos of the past in the picture frames of your home. Instead get new visions in your frames and see yourself accomplishing what is in those frames. It is time to pick yourself up, dust yourself off and believe again.

I believe what you read throughout these pages can change your life. It isn't knowledge that will change your life, but applied knowledge that will cause true transformation. We are in this together. Not one of us can do this alone. I would like to be your friend, a source of help or a shoulder to lean on when the going gets tough, because it will, and we will need each other. Would you allow me the honor to be your accountability partner through the challenges and storms of life? Together, we can shine even brighter!

Are you ready to step out of the boat and into the unknown waters? Are you ready to connect so intimately with your Bodyguard that walks on water and calms the winds? Are you [really] ready to hear the heart of God and what He has for you and why on earth He created you? He is not trying to keep any mysteries from you, in fact He cannot wait to reveal them to you! Are you ready to get comfortable with being uncomfortable? Get ready to stretch in all ways possible to become the glorious being that God created you to be! You must say, "Yes to the stretch!" Together we will get back our joy, peace, balance and freedom! Are you ready? No, I mean are you truly ready for transformation?! Great I was hoping so! Take my arm as we grab a hold of Him and let's do this together! My spirit leaps that we are journeying together!

Whether your goal is to deepen your walk with Christ, begin your yoga journey, deepen your practice or become an internationally recognized yoga trainer, this book will serve all of these purposes.

I am always here for you.

In Him,

Michelle Thielen

"IF AT FIRST YOU DON'T SUCCEED, DUST YOURSELF OFF AND TRY AGAIN, YOU CAN DUST IT OFF AND TRY AGAIN."
~ Aaliyah

HOW TO USE THIS BOOK

Stretching Your Faith will guide you through a spiritual and physical practice, uniting faith and yoga. This book can be used by anyone to incorporate a physical element into their worship.

Use *Stretching Your Faith*:
- as a manual to compliment your yoga teacher training.
- to deepen your personal practice.
- to grow as a yoga teacher.
- to create intimacy with Christ.
- to strengthen your relationship with God and others.
- learning how to leave a legacy.

On these pages you'll find postures organized into eight asana families. Asana refers to postures and is used interchangeably throughout these pages. The eight asana families are categorized as; Seated, Restorative, Supine, Standing, Back Bending, Revolved, Inversions and Arm Balancing. Be sure to warm up the entire body before beginning any physical activity to avoid injury as well as achieve success and enjoyment in the postures.

Benefits and cautions of each asana family are described in the section introduction. The first posture in each chapter lists important preparatory postures designed to warm specific areas in the body before practicing the highlighted pose. The first pose also includes important counter poses designed to release the body safely or continue into a deeper posture now that you have accomplished the highlighted pose. Preparatory and counter poses are an important part of any practice. Although not listed for every posture, be sure to create your own preparatory and counter poses for a posture or series of postures known as a sequence. For example: If the highlighted pose is a hip opener, be sure to warm the hip area up before practicing the actual pose. After concluding the highlighted pose you will also want to practice counter poses to release the hips safely and effectively so that you may enjoy the full benefits of your asana practice.

Every posture includes instructions for getting into the pose, as well as suggestions to modify or deepen the pose. A posture index is included at the back for quick reference.

The Word of God is woven through these pages, helping you to understand the, often misunderstood, theories of yoga in the light of the Truth. You'll dig into the word with passages from the Bible used as your meditation which is perfectly paired with each asana family. When you see, "*Dig into the Word, Soul Work*" (not home work), this is your opportunity to get closer to the heart of God. Combined with a specific posture of prayer as you meditate on His word, your prayer life will reach to new heights that you have never experienced before. *Stretching Your Faith* will expand your worship and your yoga practice with practical applications of God given movements.

Please heed the cautions in your own practice and in your work as a yoga teacher. This book is not to be used as a medical recommendation. Please discuss your yoga practice with a physician before practicing these postures. Many postures have been known to be therapeutic or even alleviate ailments, but are not a universal solution for all. For example; Seated Pigeon has been known to be therapeutic and relieve the symptoms of sciatica. However, you may suffer from severe sciatica and Seated Pigeon is not possible for your physical limitations.

Always listen and honor you body, mind and spirit. Never force your practice, movement or postures. If your spirit needs rest, honor that. If you have an injury, be mindful to honor this. As with Christ, *Stretching Your Faith* is a journey, embrace it and enjoy basking in His presence.

To enjoy your 90 minute, 3 class instructional video, visit YogaFaith.org/GetStretched, use code SonWorshipper

WHAT IS YOGA?

Yoga, in its simplest definition is union, unite, or to yoke. Union, as it pertains to yoga, is a fusion between the mind, body, and spirit. It is a system of physical and mental disciplines that includes postures, breathing exercises, and meditation. Yoga is a personal journey where one can find balance, peace, wellness, and in YogaFaith, complete wholeness- mind, body, spirit, and soul, through Jesus Christ. A multitude of philosophical ideas has been developed by looking into the deeper dimensions of the physical, mental, and spiritual aspects of our bodies. The philosophy of yoga is the mind, body, and spirit connection, bringing oneness to our conscious and subconscious states. This is why it is unique when compared to other physical activities or exercise regimens. In YogaFaith, we speak of oneness with Christ. We look to Him for wholeness, in all dimensions of our mind, body, spirit, and soul.

In YogaFaith, the Bible is our True North; we believe what the Word of God says. The moment we receive Christ as our Lord and Savior, we receive His righteousness, power, and grace. Therefore, we are united or yoked together with Him, and the Holy Spirit dwells in us, guiding us through life. We become one with Jesus, the Father, and the Holy Spirit. Our spirit becomes perfect with His spirit. We can never lose this standing or become separated from Him. He promises to never leave or forsake us. Isn't this amazing news?

What is commonly referred to as "yoga" in the Western world can be more accurately described by the Sanskrit word "asana," which refers to the practice of physical postures or poses, commonly known as Hatha Yoga. In YogaFaith, postures, breathing, meditating and moving were created as an act of worship.

For in Him we live and move and have our being. Acts 17:28

Based on this scripture, we are moving to say thank you. "Thank you for the precious gift of life, breath, health, and abilities. I come before You with praise and thanksgiving with my whole self: body, mind, soul and spirit." This is the essence of YogaFaith.

Asanas, or postures, are a large part of yoga, but yoga incorporates more than just postures. Other important factors of yoga are breath work, meditation, balance, a state of well being, lifestyle, nutrition, and finding wholeness as we unite mind, body, and spirit with our Maker. As typical yoga is a union of the breath and postures working together, YogaFaith is a union of our movements, an act of worship, and yoking to the Lord. It is prayer in motion. It is responsive praise. While many people believe that yoga is just stretching, it is really about creating balance in the body to develop strength and flexibility. Yoga fuses together postures that have specific benefits, as well as breathing techniques and meditation, or simply a time of stillness. In YogaFaith, these things work together for His glory, and to glorify Him through our healthy, glorious temple.

Postures can be done quickly in succession, creating heat in the body through movement, also known as Vinyasa Yoga, or more slowly, to increase stamina and perfect the alignment of the body in a pose. Yoga teaches us to have balance on and off our mats. You will learn how to unite your practice of postures to balance in your everyday life.

When we become whole, our lives become whole. Only then can we help others become healed and whole. Maya Angelou said it best, "When we learn, we teach."

HISTORY OF YOGA

Yoga is a universal practice that dates back 5,000 years or more. Yoga was created in India to improve physical and spiritual health. Yoga is not a religion, nor do you have to be religious to practice yoga. Yoga does not "belong" to any individual, group of individuals, or religion, but has been practiced by individuals, groups, and organizations, as well as practiced by various religions and incorporated into traditional ceremonies.

The exact history and origin of yoga is uncertain. Evidence of yoga postures dating back to 3000 B.C. were found on artifacts and at archeological sites in the Indus Valley. Evidence of yoga was found in the oldest existing text, the Rig-Veda. Subjects in the Rig-Veda include prayer, divine harmony, and an overall greater being and wellness. Originally, yoga focused on understanding the world and others, but the Eastern world would later alter some techniques to focus on self-enlightenment.

In the 6th century, B.C., poses and meditation became an important addition in seeking self-enlightenment. Indian gurus brought yoga to the United States in the 19th and early 20th centuries. It wasn't until the 1960s that yoga increased in popularity because of its numerous benefits. In the 1980s, the Western world fully embraced the practice of yoga postures, known today as Hatha Yoga. Yoga has never been more popular than it is today, as we discover more benefits. There is a reason that over 20 million people enjoy and improve their lives by incorporating yoga into their daily lives.

In the Middle Ages (500-1500 A.D.), variations and practices stemmed off from the common Hatha Yoga practice. Bhatki Yoga is one of these stems. It focuses on surrender to God. Unlike other types of yoga, Bhatki is a spiritual journey and devotion to the divine, in our case, Jesus Christ. This is where things may get muddy for Christ followers who question practicing yoga. Hindus incorporated Bhatki yoga and other yoga techniques into their religious practices. Other religions have done the same thing. However, because Hinduism is the most popular religious group to incorporate and use yoga, some believe that yoga is Hinduism and that you have to worship their gods and philosophies in order to practice yoga. This would be like saying our Bible scriptures cannot be read by any other person, or a person of a different faith. This is what I would call "small thinking in a selfish small world, by a small god," and our God is a big God. He cannot be put into a box saying, "This was created for them, and this is created for you; this creation is for this group and you cannot have that. This Bible is only for this religion." It sounds silly, doesn't it? He is the Creator, who created things for us to enjoy. Remember, we cannot judge why or how others use yoga; the hope is that they would reciprocate the same for you and me.

YOGA DOES NOT "BELONG" TO ANY INDIVIDUAL, GROUP OF INDIVIDUALS OR ANY RELIGION

PLACE YOUR LIFE BEFORE GOD

I love how *The Message* reads Romans 12:2:

So here's what I want you to do, God helping you: Take your everyday, ordinary life—your sleeping, eating, going-to-work, and walking-around life—and place it before God as an offering. Embracing what God does for you is the best thing you can do for Him. Don't become so well adjusted to your culture that you fit into it without even thinking. Instead, fix your attention on God. You'll be changed from the inside out. Readily recognize what He wants from you, and quickly respond to it. Unlike the culture around you, always dragging you down to its level of immaturity, God brings the best out of you, develops well-formed maturity in you.

It doesn't matter what we do, or where we do it. If we are glorifying our Heavenly Father, and what we do aligns with His Word, then we have nothing to worry about. It comes back to our intentionality and what we meditate on.

Some yoga classes focus on self-enlightenment, the universe, and "self" as the light and source. Does this mean you can't attend them? This is a personal preference, but look back at Romans 12:2. Whatever we do is to glorify Him and set our hearts so they stay on Him. What if we believed that we had to be Brazilian to take a Zumba class? Do we question taking a martial arts class by asking first if we have to believe as Buddhists do to take the class? When we take a kick boxing class, typically our intention is to get healthy and fit. We don't ask to absorb what the creator's intentionality with kick boxing was when punching and kicking with fury was designed. We just go and enjoy the many benefits. We could be washing the dishes, kicking and punching the air, or stretching our bodies; it is all for His glory.

YogaFaith always dwells on the Creator, Jesus Christ, as the One True Source. If you find yourself in a class that wants your focus to turn to "self," then divert your thoughts to Him, a scripture, or a mantra such as, "Less of me and more of You God." No matter where we are or what we are doing, turning our hearts and thoughts on Him is our meditation. He is the center of everything in our lives.

YOGA + FAITH

The practice of yoga is the only form of exercise that encompasses the whole body. What I mean by the whole body is not just the physical body, but also the mind (intellect, emotions), and the spirit. The Hebrew word "Nephesh" defines the word spirit as breath, soul, and life. The definition of yoga is to unite or yoke. Yoga unites our physical practice with our mind and spirit. Remember, spirit means breath itself, soul, and life. Throughout scripture, Christ tells us to be yoked to Him and to one another. In combining our physical bodies, minds, and spiritual beings to the practice called yoga, we essentially yoke our entire spirit to Christ. His presence is as close to us as our next breath. We simply praise Him with the very breath (spirit) that He gave us. It is our way of thanking Him and praising Him in return.

There are many misconceptions of yoga, as well as many myths regarding yoga traditions. Yoga is a philosophy; it is not a religion, nor do you have to be religious to practice yoga. Yoga is nonsectarian and has the ability to deepen anyone's faith. However, in YogaFaith, our intention and heart is set on Christ Jesus. We believe He is the only way to the Father and Heaven, as John 14:6 reads:

Jesus answered, "I am the way and the truth and the life.
No one comes to the Father except through me."

There is no shortage of opinions regarding Christians who practice yoga. My hope is that you can read these pages and know the true definition of yoga; forget any preconceptions, myths, or disbelief. The enemy will try to snatch anything and everything that is good and try to bring it into darkness, but the devil is a liar!

WHAT IS YOGA?

The thief comes only to steal and kill and destroy.
I came that they may have life and have it abundantly. John 10:10

Yoga is a wonderful practice for many reasons. Daily, scientists and doctors discover more about yoga's benefits. Today, yoga is the preferred recommended therapy for hundreds of diseases, limitations, traumas, and illnesses. It is also a way to silence the chaos and distractions of our everyday lives and come back to hearing God's still small voice. Let me also remind you that the enemy wants to kill, steal, and destroy. Being made whole, healed, healthy, alive, awakened, able to change the world and increase the Kingdom is not what the enemy wants you to do, ever.

HEALTH BENEFITS

The health benefits of yoga are numerous. Studies show it can relieve symptoms of many common and potentially life-threatening illnesses such as arthritis, fibromyalgia, arteriosclerosis, chronic fatigue, diabetes, HIV/AIDS, asthma, high blood pressure, obesity, and the list goes on. A fraction of the specific benefits in physical, mental, and spiritual health are listed here. Whether you are new to yoga or have been practicing for a length of time, you will continue to learn, feel, and see the innumerable benefits of yoga.

Jesus traveled throughout the region of Galilee, teaching in the synagogues and announcing
the Good News about the Kingdom. And He healed every kind of disease and illness.
Matthew 4:23 New Living Translation

MENTAL BENEFITS

Calmness

All yoga techniques: postures, breathing techniques, meditation, and times of stillness will bring calmness to your daily life. The more one practices these techniques the more centered, balanced, peaceful and calm one will be.

Do not be anxious about anything, but in every situation,
by prayer and petition, with thanksgiving, present your requests to God. Philippians 4:6

Stress Reduction

Physical activity in general is great for relieving stress. Yoga encourages us to focus on the moment and be present as we practice, which will assist in not focusing on worries, anxieties, or stress. God promises abundant life, not a stressed out, barely-getting-by life.

Body Awareness

Like most physical activity, yoga will increase your body awareness and create overall well being. Yoga may help you realize how your body works and functions. The yoga lifestyle eventually becomes more apparent and will lead to a better self-awareness and self-confidence in all areas of your life. You will want to fuel your temple with only the best ingredients and to honor Christ in a temple that shows others just how good He is.

PHYSICAL BENEFITS

Flexibility

Yoga increases the range of motion in muscles and joints. The more you practice, the more flexible you will be. You may also take your practice into a warm or hot studio, which will increase your flexibility even more rapidly. If you practice in the hot room, use caution and don't overstretch in the heat. Younger children should also use caution in heated rooms, as their sweat glands may not be fully developed.

Strength

Many yoga postures require you to support your own body weight, which can produce great strength. Moving in and out of postures will also build stamina, strength, and endurance.

Muscle Tone

Yoga helps shape long, lean muscles. As you become stronger, you will see an increase in muscle tone.

Pain Management

Increased flexibility and strength help prevent aches and pains. Yoga greatly improves alignment and strengthens bones, which will prevent pain.

Breathing

Our natural breath is usually shallow, and uses only a fraction of our lung capacity. Pranayama, or breathing techniques, will train you to use more of your lung capacity, which benefits the entire body. Certain types of breath can also calm the central nervous system, which has both physical and mental benefits over time. Increasing our lung capacity helps us to live a longer life, and Christ died to give us an abundant, long, and prosperous life!

SPIRITUAL BENEFITS

Yoga will help you cultivate peace with yourself, others, and God. It can be a spiritual experience no matter what a practitioner's faith is, or is not. Most yoga practitioners evolve into optimistic and positive individuals through their yoga journey, incorporating the yoga lifestyle, in and out of the classroom and into every area of life. Yoga itself is nonsectarian; it promotes health and harmonious living.

I am grateful that YogaFaith has made its way into your hands. For years, a devoted community has been experiencing the power of Christ, and His healing hands working through the physical practice of YogaFaith. I believe yoga is a gift from God. The enemy will try to manipulate and turn everything that is good into darkness. I pray that you open your heart and fully surrender to the Lord, whether in a restorative posture on your mat, or while you are standing in line at the grocery store. In everything we do, we do it for His glory (1 Corinthians 10:31). Whether we are lifting weights or taking a Zumba class, He tells us to honor our temples (1 Corinthians 6:20, 1 Thessalonians. 4:4). The world may have given us misconceptions and lies about many things, including yoga and yogic techniques. My prayer is that you turn your heart and thoughts to the Lord at all times, no matter what you are doing. We don't have to be a Buddhist to practice martial arts; we don't have to be Hindu to practice yoga, and we do not have to be Brazilian to do Zumba. Just as the Bible is not just for Christians, we would not be Christ-like if we told people of other religions, "You cannot read my bible." God created us, and every good and perfect gift is from Him. Let's love one another and share healing techniques, benefits, and our great, big God with all the world!

BRANCHES OF CLASSICAL YOGA

I would be failing you if we did not review the classical branches of yoga. Some may want to know tradition, but others, not so much. We will briefly explore the branches and system of Patanjali, an Indian teacher who gathered and systematized the teachings of yoga and meditation. It is important to note that he gathered and systematized, rather than invented or created. He is believed to have lived between 200 B.C. and 450 C.E. He is the author and teacher who composed the small Sanskrit volume of *The Yoga Sutras*, from which the modern practice of yoga is derived.

In Patanjali's *Yoga Sutras*, the eightfold path is called *ashtanga*, which means "eight limbs." These eight steps act as guidelines on how to live a meaningful and purposeful life. Just as, for Christians, the Ten Commandments act as guidelines, these eight limbs serve as a prescription for moral and ethical conduct and self-discipline. They direct attention toward one's health, the world around us, others, as well as help us acknowledge the spiritual aspects of our nature.

	THE EIGHT LIMBS		
1	yama	[ya-ma]	observances of others
2	niyama	[ni-ya-ma]	self impose disciplines
3	asana	[ah-sa-na]	posture
4	pranayama	[prah-nah-yah-ma]	control of life force, breath
5	pratyahara	[pra-tyah-hah-ra]	withdrawal of the senses
6	dharana	[d-hah-rah-na]	concentration
7	dhyana	[d-hee-ah-na]	meditative absorption
8	samadhi	[sam-ahd-hi]	ecstasy

THE EIGHT LIMBS, THE TEN COMMANDMENTS, AND GOD

The first limb is known as *yama*. It breaks into another five characteristics that we will briefly touch on. Yama is associated with how we relate to the external world and others. It prepares us to be ethical and kind.

Ahimsa is the first characteristic focus of yama. It is defined as being non-violent, inflicting no injury or harm to others, or even to one's own self. It also describes that there is to be an absence of violence in thought, word, and deed. It is about us doing everything we do toward any living being with thoughtful consideration. It is a concept that all living beings have the spark of the divine in them. This is the yoga world attempting to describe what the Bible told us before there was a practice of yoga. Ecclesiastes 3:11 says that God has [already] set eternity in our hearts. Yes, we have the Divine in us! It is the power of the Holy Spirit residing on the inside of each of us. We are one with Christ.

Through the power of the Holy Spirit who lives within us,
carefully guard the precious truth that has been entrusted to you. 2 Timothy 1:14

Jesus said these words; "Love the Lord your God with all your heart
and with all your soul and with all your mind and with all your strength.
The second is this: Love your neighbor as yourself.
There is no commandment greater than these." Mark 12:29-30

Ahimsa is thought to be the most important branch, as it relates to every part of our internal and external worlds. It is the essentials: how we treat other beings, how we treat our own bodies and minds, how we think and what we think about, how we talk, what we talk about, how we eat and what we eat.

Satya is the second characteristic of the first limb. It is associated with truth in word and thought. It is about honesty and healthy relationships. Satya is defined as speaking the truth. We want to act and speak honestly, but we do not want to hurt others. Knowing when to be quiet and reserve the truth is just as important. Everything should be done in a way that we help others in some way. Ask yourself before making a decision, "Am I stealing from someone? Will my actions improve or benefit those around me? Does this thought, word, or deed harm or take away from others?" Read Hebrews 13.

...And you will know the truth, and the truth will set you free. John 8:32

It is not the truth that sets us free; the truth we *know* will set us free. There is a big difference! This is why it is important to spend time with God. Seek Him and what He wants to say to you, because this is always truth. Do you need truth or clarity? Read His Word. This is His truth, love letter, and promises to His kids! That is you and me, friend!

I am the way and the truth and the life.
No one comes to the Father except through me. John 14:6

This is one of the most important scriptures today. There is much spiritual advice that tells us that all paths lead to the same god. If you believe the Word of God, which I think you do, we can refute what the world and media tries to pour into our spirits. My Bible says there is only one way to the One True God. It is through His son Jesus. The only way that we will spend eternity in Heaven is to accept Jesus as our personal Savior.

Asteya is the third characteristic in the first limb. It is associated with not coveting, to the extent that one should not even desire something that is his own. It means to not steal, take, or use anything that has not been freely given to you. It also regards using things and information properly, not abusing or mishandling items or words that someone has confided in us.

Watch out! Be on your guard against all kinds of greed;
life does not consist in an abundance of possessions. Luke 12:15

But sexual immorality and all impurity or covetousness must not even
be named among you. Ephesians 5:3

You shall not go about as a slanderer among your people, and you are not to act against the life of your neighbor. Leviticus 19:16

THE EIGHT LIMBS, THE TEN COMMANDMENTS, AND GOD

Brahmacharya is the fourth characteristic. It refers to abstinence, particularly in the case of sexual activity. It implies celibacy, but it asks that we use our sexual energy for a connection to our spiritual side, using this energy positively and productively. Also, it calls for responsible behavior with respect to moving toward the highest truth in our relationships and ourselves. Abstinence creates the highest truth. Nothing is muddied or confused by sexual behaviors. Before a thought progresses to an action, ask if the action is betraying any of your relationships, values, principles, promises, or commitments.

And in your knowledge, self-control, and in your self-control,
perseverance, and in your perseverance, godliness... 2 Peter 1:6

Instead we should write to them, telling them to abstain from food polluted by idols,
from sexual immorality, from the meat of strangled animals and from blood. Acts 15:20

There's more to sex than mere skin on skin. Sex is as much a spiritual mystery as a physical fact. As written in Scripture, "The two become one." Since we want to become spiritually one with the Master, we must not pursue the kind of sex that avoids commitment and intimacy, leaving us lonelier than ever—the kind of sex that can never "become one." There is a sense in which sexual sins are different from all others. In sexual sin, we violate the sacredness of our own bodies, these bodies that were made for God-given and God-modeled love, for "becoming one" with another. Or didn't you realize that your body is a sacred place, the place of the Holy Spirit? Don't you see that you can't live any way you please, squandering what God paid such a high price for? The physical part of you is not some piece of property belonging to the spiritual part of you. God owns the whole works. So let people see God in and through your body.
1 Corinthians 6:16-20 The Message

The fifth characteristic is known as *Aparigraha*. It relates to freeing ourselves of possessions, hoarding stuff, or having an excess of things we do not need or no longer use. It also relates to things we have or keep what we received dishonestly, or things that we have through non-trusting or wrong methods. To sum it up: take only what is necessary. Do not exploit others, and don't hang onto things you no longer need. It implies living simply. We live in an all-consuming culture. We have pressures daily to "get" and gather more. The characteristic of a yogi and a Christian is to live a minimalistic and simple lifestyle. There is nothing wrong with "stuff;" just don't let "stuff" control you. To help with the process of becoming more simple, ask yourself if an item is truly necessary in your life. This world is in great need of what we take for granted every day. Beyond the necessities like water, food, and shelter, we have closets full of clothes and garages full of junk we don't use. Do we need all those winter coats when others are cold on the streets? And why do we pack and move all of our stuff that we no longer use, taking it from garage to garage? Aparigraha is trusting God to provide for you every day.

Look at the birds of the air; they do not sow or reap or store away in barns,
and yet your heavenly Father feeds them. Are you not much more valuable than they?
Matthew 6:26

So put to death the sinful, earthly things lurking within you.
Have nothing to do with sexual immorality, impurity, lust, and evil desires.
Don't be greedy, for a greedy person is an idolater, worshiping the things of this world. Colossians 3:5

The second limb of the eight-fold is *Niyama*, or personal observances. They are more intimate and personal than the first limb. Practicing these disciplines is more about living from the soul. The five observances include how we relate to ourselves (inner world), self-discipline, and spiritual observances.

First observance is *Sauca*, which means cleanliness of body and mind. Yoga postures cleanse and purify our physical bodies. Breathing techniques cleanse our lungs and bodily systems, and meditation on the Holy Spirit cleanses us inside and out. This discipline is being free from junk, whether physical, mental, emotional, spiritual, or in relationships. We must cleanse our bodies and minds daily. Our hearts have to be cleansed of hatred, unforgiveness, anger, bitterness, and any other negative emotions. It is always an "inside job." God always begins within us.

First wash the inside of the cup and the dish, and then the outside will become clean, too. Matthew 23:26

Do not conform to the pattern of this world, but be transformed by the renewing of your mind.
Then you will be able to test and approve what God's will is—His good, pleasing and perfect will. Romans 12:2

The second observance is *Santosa*, defined as contentment, and being satisfied with what we have. This is about being happy with what we have and what we do not have. This discipline is about having joy, no matter what circumstances surround us. Yes, I'm calling it a discipline because having joy amidst trials does not always come naturally. As Christians, we know that all things work together for the good for those that love Him, so we count everything towards His glory. He promises to give us double for our trouble! So we can rest at all times, knowing that He has it all figured out. Isn't this wonderful news? All we [ever] have to "do" is rest and trust.

THE EIGHT LIMBS, THE TEN COMMANDMENTS, AND GOD

You satisfy me more than the richest feast. I will praise You with songs of joy. Psalm 63:5

Consider it pure joy, my brothers and sisters, whenever you face trials of many kinds, because you know that the testing of your faith produces perseverance. Let perseverance finish its work so that you may be mature and complete, not lacking anything. If any of you lacks wisdom, you should ask God, who gives generously to all without finding fault, and it will be given to you. But when you ask, you must believe and not doubt, because the one who doubts is like a wave of the sea, blown and tossed by the wind. That person should not expect to receive anything from the Lord. Such a person is double-minded and unstable in all they do. James 1:2-8

The next discipline is *Tapas*, which means to discipline the use of our energy. It relates to austerity and is associated with body and mind discipline. Tapas refers to keeping a sound mind as well as keeping our body fit with physical activity and proper nutrition. This is a discipline of controlling our inner urges so the exterior shows our disciplined lifestyle and ultimately glorifies God.

No discipline is enjoyable while it is happening-it's painful! But afterward there will be a peaceful harvest of right living for those who are trained in this way. Hebrews 12:11

The fourth observance *Svadhyaya*, relates to any self-study or self-examination. Knowing God and the soul leads to a great awakening as to how God created us to live. Sometimes we simply need a check-up from the neck up! It is important to know what's going on internally. If we don't check in and find resolution, we eventually explode, quite often toward the people near and dear to us. Daily renew your mind and "check in." Make an appointment with yourself to get quiet and find solutions to anything that may be brewing or unresolved.

Wake up, my soul, wake up, lyre and harp! I will awaken at dawn. Psalm 57:8

Do you not know that you are God's temple and that God's Spirit dwells in you? 1 Corinthians 3:16

The last observance is *Isvarapranidhana*; the definition means to lay all your cares at the feet of God. It is an act of surrender to God, surrendering everything, all of it. Give all your cares to Him.

I'm speaking in a human way because of the weakness of your corrupt nature. Clearly, you once offered all the parts of your body as slaves to sexual perversion and disobedience. This led you to live disobedient lives. Now, in the same way, offer all the parts of your body as slaves that do what God approves of. This leads you to live holy lives. Romans 6:19 God's Word Translation

Give me your heart, and let your eyes observe my ways. Proverbs 23:26

Let us draw near with a true heart in full assurance of faith, with our hearts sprinkled clean from an evil conscience and our bodies washed with pure water. Let us hold fast the confession of our hope without wavering, for He who promised is faithful. Hebrews 10:22-23

The third limb, *Asana*, is defined as seat, and is used interchangeably with posture and pose. It refers to any of the postures used in yoga for the purpose of achieving balance, promoting physical and spiritual health, and attaining mental calmness.

FOR IN HIM WE LIVE AND MOVE AND HAVE OUR BEING. Acts 17:28

Don't you realize that all of you together are the temple of God and that the Spirit of God lives in you? 1 Corinthians 3:16

Or didn't you realize that your body is a sacred place, the place of the Holy Spirit? Don't you see that you can't live however you please, squandering what God paid such a high price for? The physical part of you is not some piece of property belonging to the spiritual part of you. God owns the whole works. So let people see God in and through your body.
1 Corinthians 6:19 The Message

The fourth limb is *Pranayama*, defined as breath, or life force. Many breathing techniques improve our overall health and well being. We can practice these for specific ailments to cleanse our bodily systems or calm our anxieties.

And to every beast of the earth and to every bird of the heavens and to everything that creeps on the earth, everything that has the breath of life, I have given. Genesis 1:30

This is what the Sovereign Lord says to these bones: "I will make breath enter you, and you will come to life. I will attach tendons to you and make flesh come upon you and cover you with skin; I will put breath in you, and you will come to life. Then you will know that I am the Lord." Ezekiel 37:5-6

The fifth limb is called *Pratyahara*, defined as withdrawing or retreating. This is a withdrawal of the senses, or a control of the senses, and directs our attention internally. It implies that we should pull away from anything that does not nourish our senses. We should withdraw from external distractions and attachments and in doing so, we conserve our focus and energy towards a higher calling. Without unnecessary distractions, our center, senses, and emotions become keenly sharpened. We become more aware, which allows us to properly discern things in our lives, and spend more time focused on the things, people, and circumstances that pertain to our destiny.

The practice of *Pratyahara* allows us to observe our habits objectively. We become aware of the daily habits that serve us, and those that no longer serve us. We can then begin to prioritize our daily activities and habits. If they no longer align with our destiny, then we do not make them a priority. We replace old, unhealthy habits with new habits that serve our purpose.
Ask yourself, "Is what I'm doing drawing me closer or further away from my destiny? Why am I doing this? What is the purpose of this activity?" Even if the thing you're doing is good, it can distract you from your true destination and ultimately be a waste of precious time. When was the last time you withdrew?

Examine me, God, and know my mind, test me, and know my thoughts.
Psalm 139:23 International Standard Version

Early in the morning, well before sunrise, Jesus rose and
went to a deserted place where He could be alone in prayer. Mark 1:35

After He had dismissed them, He went up on a mountainside by Himself to pray.
Later that night, He was there alone. Matthew 14:23

The sixth limb is called *Dharana*, which is defined as an immovable concentration of the mind. It means to focus, dwell, meditate, and think upon a singular thing. This is meditation at its deepest level, being completely engrossed and focused on one thing, not several fleeting thoughts at one time. B.K.S. Iyengar founder of Iyengar yoga, states that the objective is to achieve the mental state where the mind, intellect, and ego are "all restrained and all these faculties are offered to the Lord for His use and in His service." Here, there is no self, only self-less. The ego dissipates, and you allow space in the innermost parts for the Holy Spirit to consume you. Exhale you; inhale Him.

Whatever is true, whatever is worthy of reverence and is honorable and seemly,
whatever is just, whatever is pure, whatever is lovely and lovable,
whatever is kind and winsome and gracious,
if there is any virtue and excellence, if there is anything worthy of praise,
think on and weigh and take account of these things [fix your minds on them]. Philippians 4:8

I do not consider myself to have embraced it yet, but this one thing I do:
forgetting what lies behind and straining forward to what lies ahead. Philippians 3:13

It will take time to reach this level of meditation. It is difficult to set aside a few moments each day, let alone many, and focus on only one thing. The one thing is God and Him alone. Allow everything else to melt away as the Spirit consumes your cares. This observance is when ultimate freedom and healing will take place so we can move from our past hurts and failures to the abundant and victorious life God has already predestined for us.

The seventh limb is *Dhyana*, which means worship or profound meditation. Simply put, it is perfect contemplation. Practice the previous observance of meditating on one thing. Here we will dive a little deeper into meditation. The seventh observance is the truth and knowledge of the One Christ we have been meditating on. We seek to understand His ways and truth. This is deep and profound meditation. It is an uninterrupted flow of concentration, or dwelling on the Lord. Here we can be keenly aware, without focus. Our mind, with its anxious thoughts and our heart, with its many worries, become quiet. It is in this stillness, where few thoughts exist and Christ can pierce our hearts, minds, and spirits; His Spirit speaks to our spirits.

But they delight in the law [the instructions] of the Lord, meditating on it day and night. Psalm 1:2

They are constantly in my thoughts. I cannot stop thinking about Your mighty works. Psalm 77:12

The eighth and final stage of ashtanga is *Samadhi*, which means absorption, bringing together, or merging. It is described as a state of ecstasy as our minds stay aware and conscious, while our bodies and senses are mostly at rest. During this stage, we can truly transcend "self" and completely connect with God. Does this give you a new definition of ecstasy, or what?! Here, you will find peace with yourself, others, all living beings, and the [true] peace that passes all understanding.

And the peace of God, which transcends all understanding,
will guard your hearts and your minds in Christ Jesus. Philippians 4:7

In YogaFaith, we set our hearts, minds, and spirits on the Lord. We never "empty" our minds. You may have heard of a yoga practice that attempts this; it is impossible to empty the mind. It can be difficult to still and quiet everything down to let go of intellect and distractions. However, as we let go of "self" and become enveloped in the Holy presence of our Father, we can experience truth, peace, and joy on the highest possible level.

No one has ever seen God. But if we love each other, God lives in us,
and His love is brought to full expression in us. 1 John 4:12

For the one whom God has sent speaks the words of God,
for God gives the Spirit without limit. John 3:34

For by these He has granted to us His precious and magnificent promises,
so that by them you may become partakers of the divine nature,
having escaped the corruption that is in the world by lust. 2 Peter 1:4

You love Him even though you have never seen Him.
Though you do not see Him now, you trust Him;
and you rejoice with a glorious, inexpressible joy. 1 Peter 1:8

THE YOGI AND CHRISTIAN LIFESTYLE

And whatever you do, in word or in deed, do everything in the name of the Lord Jesus,
and let it be through Him that you give thanks to God the Father. Colossians 3:17

"WHEN YOU DO SOMETHING, DO IT WITH ONE HUNDRED PERCENT OF THE MIND. DON'T DO IT HALF WAY. WHATEVER YOU DO, DO IT WITH FULL CONCENTRATION. THAT IS YOGA."
-Swami Satchidananda

The yoga and Christian lifestyle include certain principles and values that parallel each other. Scripture tell us that in whatever we do, do it all for His glory (1 Corinthians 10:31). We have studied the Eight Limbs which are the foundation of yoga's traditional guidelines toward a harmonious lifestyle, we will further explore the five characteristics of the first limb. Within these classical eight limbs of yoga, we see essential similarities to the word of God and will dive deeper into what God's Word says about the way we are to live, how we are to treat others, as well as how we are to extend our many blessing and gifts with the world we live in.

These are basic guidelines for the yogic lifestyle. The very essence of yoga is unity, as we know it's definition is to "yoke". God tells us to give Him our heavy burdens that we were never meant to carry and exchange it for His yoke, which is light. (Matthew 11:30) When we receive Christ as our Lord and Savior, we are yoked together with Him. He dwells within us. Just like any of our relationships, the more time we spend with a person the more we get to know them intimately. Christ longs to spend time with us. He asks us to "draw near" and in return He draws nearer to us. (James 4:8) The key to knowing Him is spending time with Him. Walking with Him, reading His promises, getting still to listen, worship and pray, as well as accepting His grace. We cannot enjoy the benefits of Him or His amazing gifts if we don't actually receive or accept them. You would never leave a gift on your porch, you must unwrap the gift to experience it. The more of ourselves we lay down to let more of Him come in, the more we will become like Him, and bear the fruits of His Spirit. Who wouldn't want to be more like Jesus?

Galatians 5 describes the fruit of the Spirit. I encourage you to study the fruits of the Spirit in depth for a life changing course. There are specific items that we must "put on" each and everyday, just as we do our physical clothes, we must clothe our spiritual body as well. Don't leave the house naked!

The fruit of the Spirit is love, joy, peace, patience, kindness, goodness, faithfulness.
Galatians 5: 22

Five Characteristics of the First Limb; Yama: Self Restraints
AHIMSA = Non-violence (Mark 12:30-31)
SATYA = Truthfulness (John 8:32, 14:6)
ASTEYA = Non-stealing (Luke 12:15, Ephesians 5:3)

BRAHMACHARYA = Faithfulness (2 Peter 1:6)
APARIGRAHA = Non-greed (Colossians 3:5)

Keep your lives free from the love of money and be content with what you have, because God has said,
never will I leave you; never will I forsake you. Hebrews 13:5

Finding inner peace and true joy is the ultimate goal of the yoga lifestyle and the by-product of following Christ. Yoga unites, or yokes, our breath with our postures. YogaFaith unites meditation, prayer, worship, and praise with our yoga practice. It is important to take what we learn on the mat and unite it with our world outside of our practice. You will take what you learn in the moments of stillness and meditation into the world around you. YogaFaith allows you to find balance, peace, joy, and wholeness in our mind, body, soul, and spirit. To enter the presence of the Almighty and receive from Him so that we can extend [Him] out.

An example of how we can begin to take our practice 'off our mat', is to think of a challenging posture. As you settle into this challenging pose, it becomes necessary to turn your focus to your breath, deepen your awareness of Christ's strength in you, and turn your focus on Him. In challenging circumstances, we can practice what we learn on our mats by taking deep inhalations and exaggerated exhalations when needed, just as we did in the posture. We can 'dig deep' and find the strength and focus that He gives us and use it all for our challenging situations that life throws in our direction. You may find yourself becoming less reactive and more pliable. Reading scriptures and ancient yoga teaching may help you to be kind to all beings, not just people. You may find yourself helping the environment more by being aware of the footprint you have and how everything you do affects another generation on planet Earth. You may find that you don't want to eat animals that were placed here to coexist and for us to enjoy. These guidelines and principles can help you find the joy and strength in the Lord that He promises to give you.

YogaFaith is about sharing your light that He gives you, your unique gifts and talents with those who cross your pathway. Often you hear Namaste at the end of a yoga class, Namaste simply means; The light in me honors the light in you. In YogaFaith we know this Light, and acknowledge the source as Christ, He is our True Source. You can think or meditate on this mantra by honoring, respecting, and being kind to those in your world. Begin to act like the One you are starting to spend more and more time with. Study Galatians 5 and meditate on the fruits of the Spirit and begin to walk those out in your everyday life.

Jesus had an open heart while walking this Earth. He graciously received interruptions and distractions as opportunities. In today's world, how many of us don't have even a little margin available because we are so busy? I'm sure you have heard that B.U.S.Y. means "Buried Under satan's Yoke." Isn't it true? When we spend time with Christ, we become more like Him as well as more available to those around us. Start looking at interruptions as opportunities to share the love of Christ. You don't even have to say His name. The time you share with Him will equate to acting like Him, which means to love people, walk in His ways, be kind to others and pray for those who curse you. (I know, ouch!) How about bless those who curse you? (Double ouch right?) Believe it or not, after spending time with your Heavenly Father, these things will become easy and become a joy to practice.

We can learn so much from others around us if we would just open our hearts up more, be willing to take time to get to know somebody we may not normally open our lives up to or by simply nurturing an existing relationship a bit more, take time, just as Jesus did. Multitasking and being busy is very overrated! Let's commit to being simply present, doing one task at a time, and becoming less busy.

I challenge you right now to "look up" more. Unplug from all your gadgets and look up so you don't miss what God is doing, or perhaps a divine connection. Your future spouse could pass you by if you're looking down! I encourage you to spend more time face-to-face and less time on Facebook. (or whatever is taking your attention from real life relations.) Let's get unbusy, unplug and look up! Multitasking is overrated!

MULTITASKING IS OVERRATED

MEDITATION

The definition of meditation is continued or extended thought, reflection, contemplation, devout religious contemplation, or spiritual introspection. *Encyclopedia Britannica* describes meditation as a private religious devotion or mental exercise in which techniques of concentration and contemplation are used to reach a heightened level of spiritual awareness.

The purpose of meditation is to ponder, create inner peace, calmness, and to connect with Christ. As followers of Christ, we know meditation is found throughout the Bible and is just as important as praying, fasting, tithing, or any other act of worship to Him. The enemy has even attempted to turn the word meditation into something dark. But scripture repeatedly tells us to meditate, or deeply ponder, the things of God.

Meditation can be difficult to begin, but it is important and transformational. A devil roams and seeks our souls, I can tell you He never wants to you find time and space for your Savior, or to know scripture and their profound truth.

MEDITATION

Begin to find quiet time to focus. Perhaps simply focus on your breath at first. Close your eyes, then begin to come into meditation, dwelling, deeply contemplating, setting your heart and intention on the Lord. In whatever we do, it is all about our intentionality.

May the words of my mouth and the meditation of my heart be pleasing to You,
oh Lord, my rock and my redeemer. Psalm 19:14 New Living Translation

May my meditation be pleasing to Him, for I rejoice in the Lord.
Psalm 104:34 English Standard Version

If our mind is stayed on Him and we have the peace that passes all understanding, then we will be free from worries and able to experience true happiness. However, if we don't spend time with God and our minds are not peaceful, it is difficult to live a happy or abundant life as He wants us to do.

The more you meditate, the closer you become to God. The closer you are to Him, the more you get to know Him, which translates in knowing His promises and His plans for your life. You will have more peace and joy just by being in His presence, which will flow into every other area of your life. This does not mean that you will have an absence of chaos, but you will know the One who can get you through the chaos.

When the storms of life come, the wicked are whirled away,
but the godly have a lasting foundation. Proverbs 10:25

Notice it says "when," not "if." It's important to spend time with God so He can equip us to handle the storms *when* they come. Getting alone with Him and meditating on His Word will help you do this. In simplest terms, meditation is contemplation. I encourage you to set aside time every day to contemplate with Christ, and watch your world begin to change!

HOW TO MEDITATE

To begin this ancient and powerful practice, find a quiet place where you can be still and free from distractions. Get into a comfortable position, where your breath can flow easily. Seated postures are recommended, but lying down is okay too. It's okay to fall asleep in the Lord's arms and presence. Close your eyes and begin to focus on calming your breath. Begin to contemplate, reflect, and accept things for what they are. Ask God what He has for you in this storm or victory. Meditation is a time to be still and find peace, purity, and joy. Begin to focus on God, a scripture, or a promise. Sometimes a simple question such as, "What brings you peace? Joy? Healing? What helps you to become the best you?" can help you get into a meditative state. You may find that it's difficult to silence voices, negative thoughts, to-do lists, or circumstances. The more you practice meditation, the easier it will become. Try to focus on your breath or the face of God. Maybe you begin to remember what the Lord has done in your life, and dwell on these things. Remember Philippians 4:8:

Whatever is true, whatever is worthy of reverence and is honorable and seemly, whatever is just, whatever is pure, whatever is lovely and lovable, whatever is kind and winsome and gracious, if there is any virtue and excellence, if there is anything worthy of praise, think on and weigh and take account of these things [fix your minds on them].

You may find it difficult to stay still for a few minutes. Try to start with a small amount of time, such as five minutes. You can work up to longer periods, and it will become easier each time, especially when you see the change in yourself from spending time in His presence. How many times do we read throughout scripture that people were transformed by His presence, even if it were a few moments? Do you want transformation? Spend time with God.

There are times when we need urgent answers from the Lord. Go to Him with those pleas and cries. Enter into His presence with praise and thanksgiving. If you are going through something specific, find scriptures related to that subject, and take those into your prayer closet to meditate. The more you meditate on His promises and Word concerning your dilemma, the more these promises are etched into your heart! Begin to speak them over your life, family, circumstance, or whatever you are praying for, and watch God do great miracles.

My mouth will speak words of wisdom;
the meditation of my heart will give you understanding. Psalm 49:3

How I love Your instruction! It is my meditation all day long. Psalm 119:97

MEDITATION

I have more understanding than all my teachers,
for your testimonies are my meditation. Psalm 119:99

But you are doing away with the fear of God and hindering meditation before God. Job 15:4

DO YOU WANT TRANSFORMATION? SPEND TIME WITH GOD.

Prayer:
Father, thank You for creating me and knowing my innermost parts. As I come to You and seek You, You fill me with Your truth and Spirit so I can be awakened to see and hear what You have for me. Thank you for carrying me through my battles and always protecting me and keeping me secure and safe. I commit to You today that I will glorify You with every breath that I take. My thoughts and meditations will stay perfectly on You, and You will continue to speak and guide me into all truths!

THE POSTURES OF PRAYER

Never stop praying. 1 Thessalonians 5:17 New Living Translation

This is our commandment: to never stop praying. Pray without ceasing. There is no right or wrong way to pray; no position of a prayer is superior to another. The only thing that we as believers must do is to humble ourselves before the Lord, acknowledge His Lordship of our lives, and pray without ceasing. The following are simply observations on prayer postures found in the Bible that may elevate your spoken prayers. At times, the postures of our prayer can let God know that we are serious about specific issues. Again, we are observing the powerful and miraculous prayers of great men and women of the Bible. If Jesus needed to get alone on His knees to pray, why would we think that it isn't important for us to do the same?

As we combine our faith with our movement, or put our "prayers in motion" with YogaFaith, we can recall ancient times and miracles as we move, breathe, and have our being (Acts 17:28). If there is an urgent request, we can find ourselves in a prone position, flat on our face before the Lord, as many were in scripture. Perhaps we find ourselves in a simple seated position to simply quiet our anxious thoughts and meditate on Him. You will read about these postures and their meaning. Keep in mind, there are no rules.

Sometimes it is not just about what we are praying, but how we are praying. The posture of our prayers can take our prayer life to a whole new level of intimacy with Christ. There is no mistaking that God hears our prayers, even if we don't speak them at all. When we are born again and receive salvation, we become one with Christ. He dwells in us. His spirit is all-consuming and envelops our every fiber. This is the time when grace piled upon grace enters into our lives. It becomes our [true] desire to live for God and cause Him to smile each day by our actions, words, deeds, gifts and talents. Even if our prayers go unspoken, God can perceive our words before they are thoughts, He knows our thoughts well before they are [actual] thoughts (Psalm 139:2). I am sure you have experienced times when you do not know what to pray. God knows what you need before you even utter a word!

The Lord knows the thoughts of man, that they are but a breath (Psalm 94:11). Sometimes when we cry, that is the only prayer needed. Often I have found the only prayer I can pray is one word, "Jesus." He knows the rest. Other times, I simply hold the Bible up to my heart in silence and download His great and precious promises. Prayer is our lifeline. Without prayer, whether spoken or unspoken, there is no communication with the Life Giver.

Throughout scripture, we see how prayer postures elevated the meaning of the spoken prayer. Regardless of any posture you pray in, the most important posture is truly the posture of your heart. Keep this in mind as you read the following posture descriptions. To say that one prayer posture is superior to another would be biblically incorrect. The bible teaches us that God loves variety, and He speaks to each of us differently. There are no rules, no right or wrong way, just as long as we pray! Always be spirit-led and never led by anything or anyone else. Because whether we are standing, sitting, kneeling, or flat out on our faces, our hearts must be humbled in acknowledging the Lordship of Jesus Christ. This is more important than any external physical position.

THERE IS NO RIGHT OR WRONG WAY TO PRAY; JUST DO IT.

Standing

Prayers that were offered while standing were for adoration, thanksgiving, worship, and praise. While standing in awe of God, the hands were typically open with the palms facing upward toward Heaven. Generally speaking, the eyes were open and lifted toward the heavens.

Orans is the Latin word for *praying with hands extended*. It is the oldest prayer posture found in scripture and most commonly used in today's western churches, Jewish synagogues, practiced during mass, and the standard position for taking communion together. Some pastors today require standing for the reading of God's Word. During this time, many lift their hands or face their palms upward to receive and absorb the words or prayers that are being spoken. Seeing a church gather and stand at the reading of God's word proves that there are Christians who honor, revere, and respect the written Word of God.

Some of the most memorable stories and miracles from the Bible have come from standing postures that look up to Jesus or Heaven.

In every place of worship, I want men to pray with holy hands lifted up to God, free from anger and controversy. 1 Timothy 2:8

Jesus spoke these things; and lifting up His eyes to heaven, He said, "Father, the hour has come." John 17:1

Then Jesus looked up and said, "Father, I thank you that you have heard me." John 11:41

The Mountain of Transfiguration, *"But I say to you truthfully, there are some of those standing here who will not taste death until they see the kingdom of God." Some eight days after these sayings, He took along Peter and John and James, and went up on the mountain to pray. And while He was praying, the appearance of His face became different, and His clothing became white and gleaming. And behold, two men were talking with Him; and they were Moses and Elijah, who, appearing in glory, were speaking of His departure which He was about to accomplish at Jerusalem. Now Peter and his companions had been overcome with sleep; but when they were fully awake, they saw His glory and the two men standing with Him.* Luke 9:27-33

I look up to the hills from where my help comes from. Psalm 121:1

Hannah presented to the Lord her petition while standing, and the Lord answered her. 1 Samuel 1:26

Stand in awe, and sin not: commune with your own heart upon your bed, and be still. Selah. Psalm 4:4

In Luke 18:10-14, *God answered the prayers of sinners as they stood, prayed, and humbled themselves. "Two men went up into the temple to pray, one a Pharisee and the other a tax collector. The Pharisee stood and was praying this to himself: 'God, I thank You that I am not like other people: swindlers, unjust, adulterers, or even like this tax collector. 'I fast twice a week; I pay tithes of all that I get.' "But the tax collector, standing some distance away, was even unwilling to lift up his eyes to heaven, but was beating his breast, saying, 'God, be merciful to me, the sinner!' "I tell you, this man went to his house justified rather than the other; for everyone who exalts himself will be humbled, but he who humbles himself will be exalted."*

One of my most beloved stories in the Bible is found in 2 Chronicles 20. It's a story of how God answered Jehoshaphat as he and his small army gathered corporately and stood in prayer, believing God would fight their overwhelming battle for them as they obeyed His commandment of standing still. God performed a miracle. Jehoshaphat and his people stood victorious in the face of their defeated enemy! When you have done all that you can do, stand!

Then Jehoshaphat stood up in the assembly of Judah and Jerusalem at the temple of the Lord in the front of the new courtyard... All Judah was standing before the Lord, with their infants, their wives and their children. 2 Chronicles 20:5, 13

So use every piece of God's armor to resist the enemy whenever he attacks,
and when it is all over, you will still be standing up. Ephesians 6:13 The Living Bible

The Message Version: *"Be prepared. You're up against far more than you can handle on your own. Take all the help you can get, every weapon God has issued, so that when it's all over but the shouting you'll still be on your feet. Truth, righteousness, peace, faith, and salvation are more than words. Learn how to apply them. You'll need them throughout your life. God's Word is an indispensable weapon. In the same way, prayer is essential in this ongoing warfare. Pray hard and long. Pray for your brothers and sisters. Keep your eyes open. Keep each others' spirits up so that no one falls behind or drops out."*

Seated

Seated prayer postures typically demonstrate one who is seeking guidance, counsel, or instruction from the Lord. Sometimes we read how one would use a seated position simply to be alone, find calm, peace, and quiet to bask in the presence of God. Jesus often went to be alone with His Father and pray. Other times, we read how one would sit to pray and let God know they were ready and willing to serve Him and walk in obedience. We may need to remind ourselves to sit quietly and bask in His presence more often, or perhaps sit down with the Lord and let Him know we are ready to walk in obedience.

Have you ever said to the Lord, "Here I am. Send me?" Perhaps it is time. Are you ready? Are you willing? Let us sit and surrender our will. Let us sit and ask for guidance. Let us sit before the Lord and tell Him we will serve Him for the rest of our days, then let us sit and ask, "Where do you want me to go, and what do you want me to do oh Lord?" He will answer you. Simply sit in His presence in stillness, and listen. Prayer is a dialogue; it is not a monologue. He speaks, and we listen. We speak, and He hears us. As with any conversation, we must be quiet and listen to Him. Seated postures are used most often for meditation. While combining our faith with yoga, these are great postures to sit quietly in His presence and converse with the Creator of the Universe, your "Dad!" Imagine climbing on your dad's lap and talking to Him. Maybe you just wrap your arms around Him and say nothing at all?

King David sat down before the Lord to inquire, "Why me Lord?" Then King David went in and sat before the Lord, and he said: "Who am I, Sovereign Lord, and what is my family, that you have brought me this far?" 2 Samuel 7:18

As I was sitting in my house with the elders of Judah sitting before me, that the hand of the Lord God fell on me there, and who is ready to serve Him. Ezekiel 8:1

Then all the Israelites, the whole army, went up and came to the house of God [Bethel] and wept; and they sat there before the Lord and fasted that day until evening and offered burnt offerings and peace offerings before the Lord. Judges 20:26 Amplified

THE POSTURES OF PRAYER

Fasting is an expression of emptying oneself out to seek the Lord so that His word, will, and presence would be the one and only thing that would fill us up. Here, and many other passages, we see the manifestation of miracles that occur when we couple our prayers with fasting. Combining a specific prayer posture with fasting can elevate the intensity of our request and petitions. It will demonstrate to God that we are serious about His call on our life.

Be still, and know that I am God! Psalm 46:10

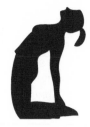

Kneeling

Kneeling is a traditional posture that demonstrates humility, repentance, submission, and supplication. It is the position we see most often where one is seeking favor or making their supplications known to God. When we practice a kneeling pose, we can acknowledge our weakness and grant His strength and power access to our every fiber. Let's use camel pose, shown as the silhouette here, as an example. This is a great kneeling back bend, but it also allows us to open our hearts upward to God. During this pose, we can surrender all and worship wholly!

And at the evening sacrifice I arose up from my heaviness; and having rent my garment and my mantle, I fell upon my knees, and spread out my hands unto the Lord my God. Ezra 9:5

Come, let us bow down in worship, let us kneel before the Lord our Maker. Psalm 95:6

He got down on his knees three times a day
and prayed and gave thanks before his God. Daniel 6:10

Acts 9:40 records the miracle of Peter praying on his knees asking God to raise the dead to life.

Peter sent them all out of the room; then he got down on his knees and prayed. Turning toward the dead woman, he said, "Tabitha, get up."
She opened her eyes, and seeing Peter she sat up.

When Paul had finished speaking, he knelt down with all of them and prayed. Acts 20:36

For this reason, I kneel before the Father. Ephesians 3:14

That at the name of Jesus every knee should bow,
in heaven and on earth and under the earth. Philippians 2:10

Moses bowed to the ground at once and worshiped. Exodus 34:8

Elijah climbed to the top of Carmel, bent down to the ground,
and put his face between his knees. 1 Kings 18:42

He [Jesus] knelt down and began to pray saying, "Father, if You are willing,
remove this cup from Me; yet not My will, but Yours be done. Luke 22:41-42

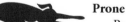

Prone

Prone (on the belly) postures typically symbolize a desperate plea, an urgent request, or to express to God complete and utter dependence on Him. There have been many times in my life when I was flat on my face desperate, or as I like to say, eating dust bunnies!

Have you ever been out of options? This is when we find ourselves flat on our faces, eating dust bunnies from the floor, and crying out to the Lord, "Save me!" Prone-positioned prayers are also used for intercessory prayers; these are typically urgent prayers in themselves. When we find ourselves grieved over a loved one or need to stand in the gap for another brother or sister, these are usually prayers of urgency and desperation. Prostrated prayers are often used for repentance and confessing sins, sometimes this is an urgent task as well. In Samuel, we see how a prone position pays honor and respect to a superior. This is also a position of true worship as we see in 2 Chronicles when Jehoshaphat bowed down face first.

Then Jehoshaphat bowed his head with his face to the ground, and all Judah and the inhabitants of Jerusalem fell down before the Lord, worshiping the Lord. 2 Chronicles 20:18

Then Joshua tore his clothes and fell to the earth on his face before the ark of the Lord until the evening, he and the elders of Israel. And they put dust on their heads. Joshua 7:6

"What does he look like?" he asked. "An old man wearing a robe is coming up," she said. Then Saul knew it was Samuel, and he bowed down and prostrated himself with his face to the ground. 1 Samuel 28:14

Then He said to them, "My soul is deeply grieved, to the point of death; remain here and keep watch with Me." And He went a little beyond them, and fell on His face and prayed, saying, "My Father, if it is possible, let this cup pass from Me; yet not as I will, but as You will."
Matthew 26:38-39

I lay prostrate before the Lord those forty days and forty nights... Deuteronomy 9:25

And all the angels stood round about the throne, and [about] the elders and the four beasts, and fell before the throne on their faces, and worshiped God. Revelation 7:11

Lying Down

Lying down and meditating on the Lord is a sweet and precious time with our Maker. Lying down, especially in bed, is a position of vulnerability and surrender. People call it Corpse Pose, but I like to call it "Resting Angel," it sounds slightly better than Corpse Pose, and is one of the most important postures in one's yoga practice. As we are on our backs, we allow the Holy Spirit to have His way in our body, heart, mind, spirit, and soul. We simply meditate on the fact that we are breathing and alive because of Him. All things are from Him, and because we were created to hear from our Creator, this is the perfect posture to do so. Allow His spirit to speak to yours. Our focus turns toward gratitude as we thank Him, spirit to Spirit, for the temples He has loaned us. This is the time to welcome stillness and a peace that passes all understanding.

Tremble and do not sin; when you are on your beds, search your hearts and be silent. Psalm 4:4

My soul is satisfied as with marrow and fatness, and my mouth offers praises with joyful lips.
When I remember You on my bed, I meditate on You in the night watches,
For You have been my help, and in the shadow of Your wings I sing for joy. Psalm 63:5-6

Moreover, the king's servants came to bless our lord King David, saying,
"May your God make the name of Solomon better than your name,
and make his throne greater than your throne," and the king bowed himself on the bed. I Kings 1:47

In peace I will lie down and sleep, for you alone, Lord make me dwell in safety. Psalm 4:8

PRAYER POSTURES QUICK GUIDE

Standing
For praise, honor, thanksgiving, worship, adoration, reverence and awe: a deep respect. A place of strength and glorifying God.

Seated
To inquire, seek counsel or guidance. Sit alone with God, and enjoy His presence. Converse and dialogue or simply meditate on your Heavenly Father. Submit, surrender, and let Him know you want to walk in obedience and serve Him.

Kneeling
Humility, submission, honor and complete surrender. Supplications and petitions made known.
Acknowledge Christ's Lordship over your life.

Prone
Urgency, emergency, humility (releasing all ego), surrender, confession, repentance, desperate pleas or cries, intercessory prayer for others or standing in the gap.

Lying Down
Resting and enjoying the presence and goodness of the Lord. Be still, quiet a busy mind and an anxious heart.
Used to meditate on Him and His precepts.

Prayer:

Dear Heavenly Father, thank You for breathing your Spirit into mine and giving me life! My praises for You shall continually be in my mouth! Today I come before You with praise and thanksgiving. I know there is no right or wrong way to pray, just that I never stop praying. There is no good, bad, correct, or wrong posture of prayer, just that we communicate with each other throughout the day. Thank You for blessing me with a healthy body, one that can practice many postures of prayer. And as I set my prayer in motion and worship You with all my heart, mind, spirit and soul, I give thanks to You for all of Your creation and what You would have me do for you while I'm here on planet earth. Thank You, Lord, for every breath. May my every breath and my healthy temple glorify You, the Living God!
In Jesus' mighty name, Amen and Amen!

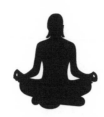

SEATED POSTURES

Be silent before the Lord and wait expectantly for Him. Psalm 37:7, Holman Christian Standard Bible

SEATED POSTURES

Let him sit alone uncomplaining and keeping silent [in hope], because [God] has laid [the yoke] upon him [for his benefit].
Lamentations 3:28, Amplified Version

In a loud and chaotic world, God is calling you. Are you able to hear His voice, or are multitudes of distractions drowning out His still small voice? He will not yell, but He is always there. Will you allow yourself time and space to come into stillness and quiet before your Maker?

YogaFaith, or "prayer in motion," is about creating time, space, and an atmosphere that welcomes your Heavenly Father "in," into every nook, cranny and fiber of your being. Throughout this journey you will experience His presence like never before as you worship with your entire mind, body, spirit, strength and soul. Yes, worship Him with everything! This is YogaFaith.

Posture or pose is also known as asana. We will use these words interchangeably. Asana is a body position, originally identified as a mastery of sitting still. In the context of yoga practice, asana refers to two things: the place where a practitioner sits and the manner (posture) in which he/she sits or stands.

Asana later became a term for various postures useful for restoring and maintaining a practitioner's well being while improving the body's flexibility and vitality. Asanas are widely known as yoga postures, positions or poses. As a collection of body and mind practices implemented through the centuries, present-day yoga is primarily sought for physical exercise. In the *Yoga Sutras*, Patanjali mentioned sitting with a steadfast mind for extended periods. Modern-day practitioners have come a long way from the original seated and meditative asana. Today, numerous styles of yoga exist, as well as a variety of postures that include sitting, standing, balancing, twisting, folding, back bending and inversions.

There are several postures in each asana family. As you practice them you may modify or deepen the postures as you desire. As you explore positions, your first priority is proper alignment and safety. *Enjoy* and *explore* the postures. They will improve as you gain strength, flexibility and mobility. After proper alignment is accomplished, you can engage the muscles and allow the posture to become active. I like to think of every muscle "hugging" the bones, unless of course, you are practicing restorative yoga. After achieving a pose, your final intent is known as *Drishti*, focus, or gaze. Focus on eliminating exterior distractions as you relax into the pose. This is where you deliberately and intentionally turn your heart and mind towards the Lord. The Bible tells us to meditate on His Word and Him, so allow your practice to be your prayers in motion and your praise in action.

Seated postures are a lovely way to spend time with God. Take time to be still, calm anxious thoughts and release tension. I encourage you to "inhale Him and exhale you" during this time together.

The mind, body and spirit all benefit from yoga postures. Seated postures help relax the whole body, which can specifically help calm the mind, provide relief from depression, stress, anxiety, tension and improve sleep issues. Seated postures are the ideal asana family to work on breath work, increasing lung capacity, opening the heart center and improving focus and mental clarity.

The spine and surrounding muscles benefit from lengthening while sitting tall, which helps release tension and increase mobility of the spine. Practicing postures that stretch and twist the spine improves posture, alignment and flexibility of the spine, while decreasing pain. Seated forward-folds and twists tone and massage abdominal organs, aid in digestion and circulation issues and calm the nervous system.

When the spine and surrounding muscles are relaxed, it's easy to release deep tension. These postures are a great way to be completely relaxed, while still present, and to focus on pranayama techniques, or breath work. Many seated postures can be therapeutic for mild cases of osteoporosis, sciatica and backache, especially in the second trimester of pregnancy. Those who suffer from limitations can usually practice several seated postures, as these poses can be gentle and can include a chair or other props that can modify the pose to accommodate almost any limitation.

Seated postures bring a sense of peace, calm and an overall sense of well being, which is the reason meditation is performed mostly in seated positions. Perhaps you can use this as your mantra: "Inhale Him and exhale me." Or choose a scripture or something that connects you with God in this intimate time you create with Him.

Benefits of seated postures include, but are not limited, to:
- Strengthening of the back muscles.
- Improving alignment of the spine, improving posture.
- Relieving backaches and pain as lumbar spine is at its natural curve.
- Improving posture as rib cage and head are rebalanced and neck becomes aligned vertically with the shoulders.
- Opening the hip and abductor muscles of the thighs.
- Increasing flexibility and lubricating hip, ankle and knee joints.
- Therapeutic for practitioners with limitations such as pregnancy, trauma, mild sciatica, backache, vertigo, glaucoma, sinusitis, osteoporosis, arthritis, AIDS, PTSD, MS, down syndrome, fibromyalgia, cancer, asthma, diabetes, heartburn and indigestion.
- Reduces stress, mild depression and anxiety.
- Improves concentration, mental focus and mental clarity.
- Relieves mental and physical exhaustion.
- Calming, renewing and restoring.

Cautions typically include, but are not limited to:
- Hip, knee or ankle injury.
- Severe sciatica, herniated disk or other major back issues.
- Pregnancy.
- Hernia.
- Diarrhea.
- Ulcers.
- Severe glaucoma, sinusitis or vertigo.

In cases of severe arthritis, sinusitis, asthma or fibromyalgia, use modifications for revolved, forward and backward bending postures. As with any posture, you may rest and hold the posture or use it in a sequence.

Dig into the Word. Your Soul Work; Ephesians 2
A Meditation for Seated Postures

THE POSTURES

SIMPLE SEATED / EASY POSE (SUKHASANA)

Simple Seated, or Easy Pose, is most often used to meditate, as your spine is supple, and full relaxation of the lungs allows for full, deep breaths. Remember Lamentations 3:28, *Let him sit alone in silence when He has laid it on him.* This is not a time to let your mind wander, but to stay active in inviting the Holy Spirit in. Settle your thoughts and focus on God, His Word and His promises. Enter into His presence with praise and thanksgiving, then make all your petitions known to Him (Philippians 4:6).

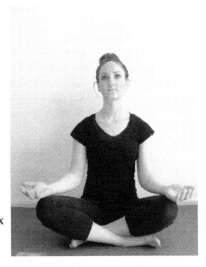

Preparatory Pose

If you would like to warm up before this posture, you can choose any hip opener such as Half Bound Lotus, Cow Posture, Cobbler's Pose, or a Reclining Bound Angle seen later in this chapter. However, you don't need to do any pose before coming into Simple Seated.

Simple Seated posture can be a great foundation and preparatory posture for all other postures, as it allows you to be still, melt tension, focus on your breath, and calm your heart. Relax into this posture. Open your heart and mind to the possibilities in your yoga practice and in life. No posture must come before, or after Simple Seated Pose.

Getting into the Posture

1. Sit comfortably on the buttocks as you cross your shins.
2. Allow your knees to rest and lengthen through the torso.
3. The outside edges of your feet connect to the earth, and rest next to the respective shin.

Modification

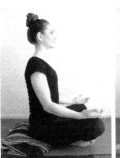

- Sit against a wall to assist with back support.
- As you inhale, focus on lengthening the spine and increasing spinal muscles.
- You may also sit on a blanket if you have lower back or hip issues.
- For a more calming position, place your palms on your knees, with the thumbs and index fingers together (Dhyana Mudra).
- You may also wrap a strap around your ankles, and gently pull on strap to focus more lengthening throughout the torso.
- For another option, press your palms together.

Blanket neutralizes
tailbone

Use a wall or
meditate here

Deepen

- Raise your arms above your head.
- Interlace your fingers, and turn your palms up.
- Close your eyes.
- Incorporate a back bend or twist from the torso side to side.
- Raise your arms, and then tilt from side to side (lateral flexion).
- You may also forward fold or recline the torso.

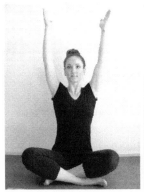
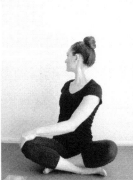
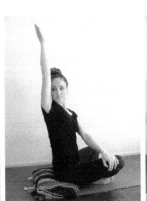
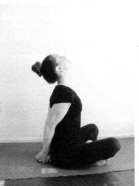
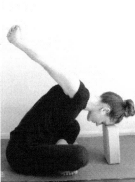

Raise arms   Add a twist   Reach and twist   Lift the heart upward   Shoulder stretch with fold

SEATED POSTURES

PERFECT POSE / SAGE (SIDDHASANA)

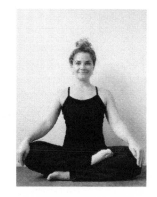

Perfect Pose is much like Simple Seated / Easy Posture, with the exception of the foot, ankle, and leg positions.

Getting into the Posture
1. Begin in Simple Seated Posture.
2. Bend your right leg, and bring your right heel to rest toward the mid line of body.
3. Allow the sole of your right foot to rest along the inner left thigh.
4. Your left heel rests in front of your right ankle.
5. Switch legs, and practice the same amount of time on opposite side.

DOUBLE PIGEON / FIRE LOG POSE (AGNISTAMBHASANA)

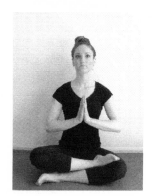

Use the same benefits, modifications and cautions as the previous seated postures. This pose allows for further opening of the hips and groin.

Getting into the Posture
1. From Simple Seated, bring one foot on top of the opposite knee.
2. The other foot is directly underneath the top leg's knee; you are stacking the ankles to knees.
3. Let your hips and groin areas relax into this posture.
4. Keep your torso lengthened and tall.
Optional: add a forward fold or a twist. Hands may rest on legs.

Counter Poses
Integrate the calming, grounded and tranquil sensations of these seated postures throughout all other postures. You may also use each one alone for times of stillness, to calm anxiety, meditate or for resting postures in the middle of any practice.

LOTUS / HALF LOTUS (PADMASANA)

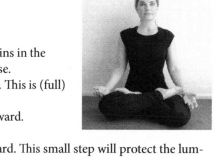

This posture can start out challenging. Just as with anything new, stick with it. Try Half Lotus first and then move into full Lotus. As you begin, inhale Philippians 4:13: I can do all things through Christ who strengthens me.

Getting into the Posture
1. From Simple Seated, bring one foot into the crease of the opposite hip, as the other leg remains in the simple seated posture, resting the outside of the foot on the earth. This is Seated Half Lotus Pose.
2. Place your other foot into the crease of the opposite hip, so both feet rest onto crease of hips. This is (full) Lotus Pose.
3. Continue to lengthen through your torso, as if a string is pulling the crown of your head upward.
4. You may add a forward fold, or come into Fish (see Deepen).
5. If coming into Fish with lotus legs, come down onto your elbows first and lift your legs upward. This small step will protect the lumbar, once your upper body achieves Fish.
6. Then relax your lotus legs back down to the earth, and enjoy this beautiful heart and hip opener.

Modification
- Sit against a wall to assist with back support. As you inhale, focus on lengthening your spine, strengthening your spinal muscles.
- You may also sit on a blanket for a more neutral pelvis, which will assist in lower back and hip issues.
- For a more calming position, place your palms on your knees, with your thumbs and index fingers together (Dhyana Mudra).
- You may also wrap a strap around your ankles. Gently pull on the strap to focus more lengthening through out the torso.
- Close your eyes, be still, and meditate on His goodness.
- You may also bring your hands to heart center.

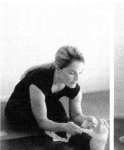 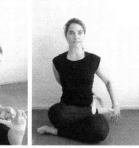 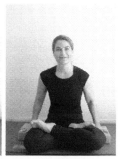

Strap around the foot or placed around the ankle   Practice with hand support

29

Deepen
- Raise your arms above your head.
- Interlace your fingers and press palms up.
- Close your eyes.
- Incorporate a back bend or twist from the torso side to side.
- Raise arms, and tilt side to side.
- May also recline posture.
- Add an arm balance by lifting the tailbone off the earth.

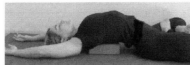

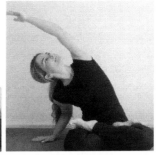

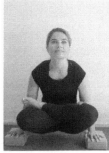

Restorative Fish with Lotus legs. Rest in Him.

Add lateral flexion

Add arm balance with blocks

To deepen further come into…

BOUND LOTUS (BADDHA PADMASANA)

Getting into the Posture
1. From Lotus, externally rotate and depress the shoulder blades.
2. Reach your opposite hand to opposite foot.

In addition to the many benefits of Lotus previously mentioned, Bound Lotus will deeply stretch your back, shoulders, and chest, as well as your throat and jaw if you gaze upward.

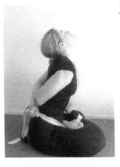

Modification
- Loop a strap around your feet and grasp at the strap until you gain flexibility to reach for your opposite foot.
- You may also simply reach for opposite elbows as well.

Focus on lengthening your spine and opening your heart to all the possibilities Christ has for you. Exhale anxiousness. Inhale peace. Exhale fear; inhale confidence.

Oh Lord, You understand my heart's desire; my groaning is not hidden from You. Psalm 38:9

To deepen further…

FORWARD FOLDING BOUND LOTUS (YOGA SEAL POSITION or YOGA MUDRASANA)

Getting into the Posture
1. From Bound Lotus, come into a forward fold. Practice with a block at your forehead in the beginning if you need to.
2. Massage your eyebrow bone from side to side on the block, or forehead if on the mat.

This pose will tone abdominal walls and greatly assist with digestion and circulation issues. Yoga Seal Pose can be therapeutic for arthritis, sciatica, osteoporosis, and menstrual and menopausal discomfort.

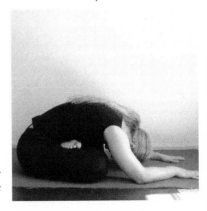

Inhalations bring in the Holy Spirit, peace, calm, and tranquility, letting your heart completely surrender. Exhalations release anything that doesn't belong in your heart and spirit. Inhale trust, and exhale insecurities in this posture.

Be silent before the Lord and wait expectantly for Him; do not be agitated by one who prospers in his way, by the man who carries out evil plans. Psalm 37:7

To modify Folding Bound Lotus, come into...

HALF BOUND LOTUS FORWARD FOLD (ARDHA BADDHA PADMA PASCHIMOTTANASANA)

With the same benefits and cautions as the previous postures, Half Bound Lotus Forward Fold is only one foot on the thigh as you forward fold. The opposite leg is bent or extended. You will continue to open the hips and knees, while stretching the spine further.

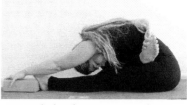

Block at foot increases reach

Getting into the Posture
1. From Simple Seated, bring one foot into the crease of the opposite hip, as the other leg remains in the simple seated posture, resting the outside of the foot on the earth.
2. Come into a forward fold.

The forward folding in these postures increase circulation to the pelvis region, and can greatly improve the digestive system as opposed to sitting straight up in these postures. To deepen your Half Bound Forward Fold, place a block at the end of foot to extend the forward fold.

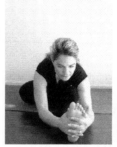 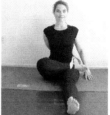

Forward fold no bind   Use a strap

Embrace your journey in this advanced posture. Exhale your doubts and worries, as you inhale true peace, balance, and serenity. What do you need to let go of? Christ wants you to surrender and release. Release everything into His care as you exhale. Fold deeper, increasing your strength for your new journey and pathway. Exhale clutter and mind chatter; inhale vitality and restoration.

God declares, "I will restore you to health and heal your wounds." Jeremiah 30:17

SEATED STAFF (DANDASANA)

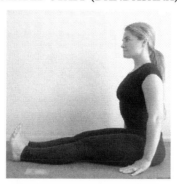

Getting into the Posture
1. Remove any excess flesh to sit directly on the sitting bones.
2. Extend your legs out in front of you, with your quadriceps facing up. Your legs are engaged and active, pressing outwardly through the heels.
3. Your spine is long, and your core is softened.

Modification
- Sit against a wall to assist with back support.
- Each inhale focuses on lengthening the spine and increasing spinal muscles.
- Sit on a blanket for a more neutral pelvis, assisting in lower back and hip issues.
- Wrap a strap around the foot (the pad as opposed to the arch) and gently pull on strap to focus more on lengthening throughout the torso.
- Keep chin and heart lifted tall.

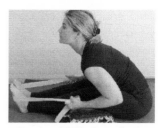

Practice with blanket and strap

Deepen
- Close your eyes, "hug tightly" the leg muscles around the leg bones.
- Incorporate a back bend, twist or forward fold.

SEATED POSTURES

SEATED FORWARD FOLD / DOUBLE LEG FORWARD FOLD (PASCHIMOTTANASANA)

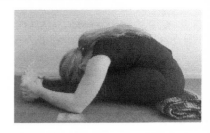

Getting into the Posture
1. From Staff Pose, lengthen through your spine.
2. Hinge forward from the hips, keeping a lengthened torso.
3. Bend your knees, or use a prop under your knees if your hamstrings are tight.
4. Flex your toes back towards your heart center.
5. Energetically rotate thighs inward so the knees are facing up.

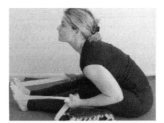

Practice with blanket and strap

Modification
- Do not forward fold, but instead sit against a wall to assist with back support.
- As you inhale, focus on lengthening the spine and increasing spinal muscles.
- You may also sit on a blanket for a more neutral pelvis, assisting in lower back and hip issues.
- Wrap a strap around your foot (the pad, as opposed to the arch), and gently pull on the strap to focus more on lengthening throughout the torso.
- Place a bolster or similar prop on top of your thighs, and then forward fold resting torso and staying elevated.

To modify further, you may also keep one knee bent and lengthen only one leg at a time coming into...

ONE LEG FOLDED FORWARD FOLD (TRIANGA MUKHAIKAPADA)

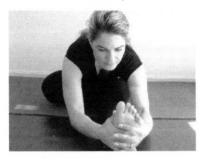

Getting into the Posture
1. From Seated Forward Fold, tuck one foot under, so you will be in Half Hero leg position with heel and buttocks close or touching. You may also use a block or cushion under the thigh and/or tailbone.
2. Continue to lengthen through your torso, hinging at the hips, while keeping your straight leg facing upward towards the sky.

Note: Inhalation will lengthen the spine and lift the heart, as exhalation lets the heart melt down towards the straight leg.

You may modify by using a strap around your foundational leg. To deepen, use a block at the bottom of your straight leg. Reach beyond your leg and grasp hands around the block.

Deepen (Seated Forward Fold, one leg or both legs)
- As you exhale, focus on deepening the posture, whatever this means to you (A deeper hinge at the hip, engaging the leg muscles more, etc.).
- Lead with your heart instead of your forehead, while your elbows melt down towards the earth.
- Flex your toes towards heart center.
- Keep the tops of your thighs facing the sky energetically.
- You may also place blocks at the soles of your feet to wrap hands further around the block and deepen the stretch.

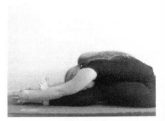

Add a block

SEATED POSTURES
SEATED OPEN A, SEATED WIDE-OPEN ANGLE (UPAVISTHA KONASANA)

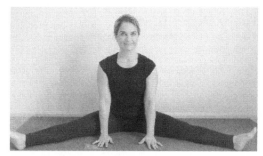

Getting into the Posture
1. From Staff Pose, separate your legs as much as you can.
2. Firmly plant your hamstrings on the earth.
3. Keep your knees and thighs facing upward.
4. Keeping your tailbone rooted down, place your hands between the thighs and slowly, begin to walk yourself down towards the earth.
5. Let your breath assist you, and lead with the heart to keep the spine as straight as possible.

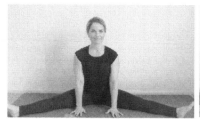
Stay upright

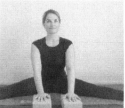
Place block under hands

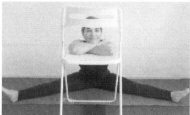
Use the seat of a chair

Modification
- Do not forward fold; instead sit against a wall to assist with back support.
- Each inhale focuses on lengthening the spine and increasing spinal muscles.
- Sit on a blanket for a more neutral pelvis, assisting in lower back and hip issues.
- Place bolster or similar prop in between your thighs, forward fold, resting torso and staying elevated.
- Stay upright, or use blocks/chair seat to rest your palms in front of you, going to your edge of the posture and breathing.
- Each inhale lengthens, and each exhale deepens your pose.

Deepen
- Each exhale will focus on deepening the posture, whatever this means to you.
- Lead with your heart instead of the forehead while walking your hands out in front of you.
- Flex your toes towards heart center.
- Keep the tops of thighs facing the sky energetically.
- Turn toward one leg; place forehead on knee.
- Keeping your legs out wide, stretch to one side.

SEATED SIDE STRETCH (PARSVA UPAVISTA KONASANA)

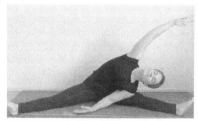
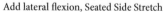
Add lateral flexion, Seated Side Stretch

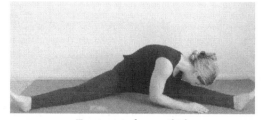
Turn torso to face one thigh

You may also like to point your toes and feel the differences between a flexed foot. Whether pointed or flexed, try to keep your thighs facing upward.

He looked around at them in anger and, deeply distressed at their stubborn hearts, said to the man, "Stretch out your hand." He stretched it out, and his hand was completely restored. Mark 3:5

Receive your healing in this posture. Exhale weakness and limitations, as you inhale restoration. To further deepen this posture, come into...

SEATED POSTURES
TURTLE (KURMASANA)

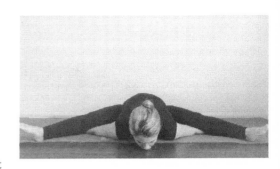

Getting into the Posture
1. Further deepening Wide A Frame Forward Fold, micro-bend your knees.
2. Tuck your arms under each knee.
3. Continue to lead with your heart as it melts down towards the earth.
4. Place your chin or forehead on the earth.
5. Continue to breathe, stretching your hands outward for a deep chest expansion. Breath is relaxed and steady.

As your heart melts into the earth, find the deepest surrender of your heart and this posture. Inhale, and lengthen the spine. Exhale, and release any insecurities. Let the Lord rejuvenate every fiber of your being! Release this stretch gently.

Further deepening the posture, come into...

RECLINING TURTLE (SUPTA KURMASANA)

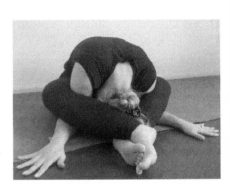

Getting into the Posture
1. From Turtle, the legs come over, on the top of your head.
2. Lock the ankles together behind or above the skull.
3. With assistance from the scapula, the hands internally rotate and slide back to the lumbar, perhaps interlocking all ten fingers.
4. Forehead, nose, and chin are on the earth.

Placing the legs behind our head has many benefits, one is that it completely invigorates our spine and all of our circulation, respiratory, lymphatic and nervous systems greatly. Keep in mind that we never know if we can do anything unless we try, and we will never achieve success unless we keep trying. Your breath will be steady and relaxed. Your exhalations will push out pride and ego, while your inhalations will bring in humility. Surrender to your deepest fears and ego. Let them all go here.

HEAD TO KNEE (JANU SIRSASANA)

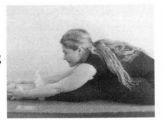

Place a block on foot at desired length to deepen stretch

Getting into the Posture
1. From Staff Pose, take one leg out to the side as you bring the opposite foot to rest on the interior of straight leg's thigh. Bending the knee or placing a cushion so that the knee is restful.
2. Root down through the tailbone, lengthen, and (slightly) rotate the torso towards the straight leg.
3. Leading with the heart center, begin to hinge from the groin area, letting your forearms down to the earth.
4. As you forward fold, belly is first, heart second, and forehead is the last part to connect as you gain flexibility.

Modification
- Lessen the forward fold.
- Place blocks or similar props under hands or forearms to keep spine elevated and keep neck neutral.
- Place blanket under knees or sitting bones.
- Use a bolster or pillow under torso.
- Use a strap around the foot of extended leg.

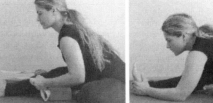
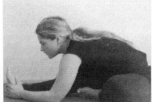
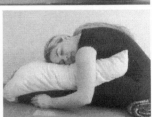

Practice with a strap and block   Lessen the hinge of forward fold   Blanket under tailbone rest on bolster or pillow

Deepen
- Each inhalation expands the rib cage slightly more and each exhalation will focus on deepening the posture.
- Flex the toes towards heart center keeping the tops of thighs facing the sky energetically. You may also like pointing the toes and feeling the differences.
- Place a block at the sole of the foot and reach around block extending the hinge. Remember to lead with your heart, the forehead is secondary and eventually connects with the knee.

You may choose another expression by coming into...

REVOLVED HEAD TO KNEE (see also Revolved Postures) (PARIVRTTA JANU SIRSASANA)

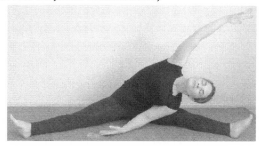

Revolved Head to Knee will further stretch the spine, shoulders, side body, and hamstrings and continue to massage and tone abdominal organs. It will greatly improve digestion and circulation issues. Try to maintain a connection between the bottom of the shoulder and the knee. When flexibility is achieved, the leg will straighten to the earth.

Revolved Head To Knee

Getting into the Posture
1. From Seated Wide A Frame, reach one hand to opposite foot.
2. Keep torso forward for a more mild twist, or turn upward for a deeper stretch.
3. The opposite arm is energetically reaching and opening the shoulder, chest and heart center.

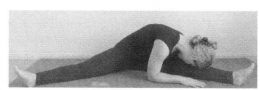

Turn torso toward leg

Modification
• Bend the opposite knee and bring foot into center.
• Only reach one arm.
• Use props or slightly turn towards leg and fold.

Deepen
• Deeply twisting the torso, both hands reach for the foot.
• Hold until fatigued.

Also try...

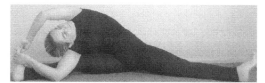

Reach both hands for foot, twisting torso

TOE STRETCHING BEYOND THE KNEE (JANU SIRSASANA C)

Getting into the Posture
1. Much like Head to Knee, with the exception of the bent leg's toe position. Place the top of the toes on the floor so the sole of the foot is on the interior of the straight leg's thigh. The heel faces upward.
2. Add a forward fold by hinging through the groin area.

In addition to the many benefits previously mentioned, this pose further opens and stretches the entire foot, hips, and knee joints greatly. It will also deepen the hamstring stretch, in addition stretch and strengthen the Achilles tendon.

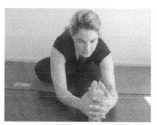

Lessen the hinge

Modification
• Lessen the hinge.
• Use a strap around the sole of the foot.
• Reach for the thigh, calf, or ankle of the straightened leg instead of the foot.

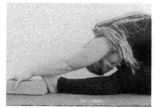

Add block for extension

Deepen
The inhalation lengthens the torso and the exhalation allows the heart to lead the torso down towards the straightened leg's shin, reaching beyond the foot or place a block on the sole of foot and reach for the block. May also add a twist to the pose.

SEATED POSTURES
BOUND ANGLE (BADDHA KONASANA)

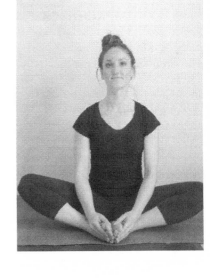

Getting into the Posture
1. Begin in Simple Seated Pose.
2. Place the soles of the feet together, using a strap around the ankles if necessary.
3. Let the interior of the feet open up like a book.
4. Root down through the tailbone as you lengthen through the spine.
5. Allow gravity to pull the knees down so the hips and groin open up to release tension.

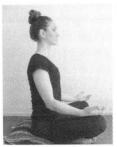

Blanket to help neutralize
the pelvis

Modification
- Sit against a wall to assist with back support.
- Sit on a high support. Each inhale focuses on lengthening the spine and increasing spinal muscles.
- Place a blanket under tailbone for a more neutral pelvis, assisting in lower back and hip issues.
- A blanket or block can also be placed under each outer thigh to relieve pressure.
- For a more calming position, place the palms down on the knees with the thumb and index fingers together (Dhyana Mudra).
- You may also wrap a strap around the ankles and gently pull on strap to bring feet closer to the tailbone.

Deepen
- Hinging at the hips, forward fold the torso in between the legs, allow the elbows to assist the knees to melt closer towards the earth.
- Another expression is to Forward Fold in your Bound Angle. Keep the torso long, hinge forward.

May also recline into the posture in...

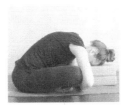 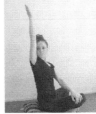 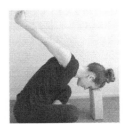

Use props   Add a twist   Arms float forward opening shoulders

RECLINING BOUND ANGLE (SUPTA BADDHA KONASANA)

Getting into the Posture
1. From Bound Angle, slowly walk your elbows behind you as you come onto your back.
2. Use props as described in modifications.

Be still in the presence of the Lord. Psalm 37:7 New Living Translation

Modification
- Lift the feet on to a block; choose the best height that suits the flexibility of your hips. The tallest height will be the most intense.
- Come into a restorative Reclining Bound Angle, use a blanket or bolster that supports the entire spine and head while blankets are underneath each outer thigh, a strap is bound around the ankles and hips, neck can have an additional support, as well as an eye pillow placed over the eyes.

Deepen
- Place a block under the sacrum or vertically between the shoulder blades, chest and/or pelvis opening up your hips and/or heart.
- Forward Fold from Bound Angle.

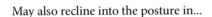

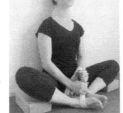 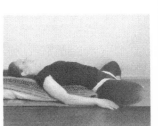

Use a wall with props   Restorative Reclining Bound Angle

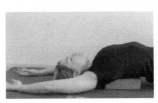 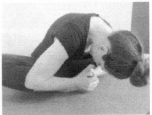

Lift your heart upward   Forward Fold

Further continuing all of the benefits from Bound Angle, is…

GRACIOUS POSE (BHADRASANA) and COBBLER / BUTTERFLY POSE (BADDHA KONASANA)

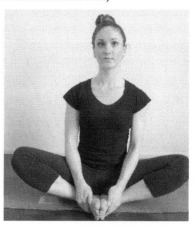

Getting into the Posture
Feet Front Gracious Pose
1. From Bound Angle, attempt to connect the heels of the feet to the perineum, while your hands hold the toes. This can be a very intense hip opener so breath remains relaxed.
2. Focus on tilting the pelvis so that the spine is stretched perpendicular to the ground, leading with the heart keeps spine straight, forward fold, or stay upright.

Deepen
- Feet go behind the body, with hips remaining wide, big toes touch near or underneath the buttocks.
- Hold until fatigued.

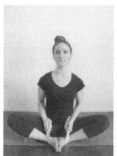
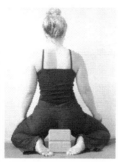
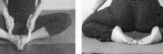

| Add strap | Gracious Pose, reverse feet | Gracious Pose, reverse feet, use blocks |

Settle in. Calm the mind. Relax the breath. Each inhalation breathes in grace and your exhalation casts out anxiety and tension.

TOE STRETCHING FORWARD FOLD (UTTHITA ANGULI SUKHASANA)

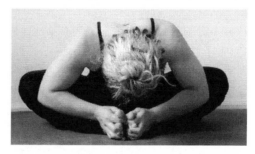

Toe Stretching Forward Fold is very much like Forward Folding Bound Angle but the elbows are on the outside of the legs as you interlace the fingers in between each toe on both feet. Because our feet are usually trapped inside shoes for most of our lives, this posture will awaken the entire foot as well as stretch and awaken the toes.

Getting into the Posture
1. Interlace all ten toes and fingers then gently squeeze all the toes.
2. Flexing the heels of the feet, the elbows come to the outside of the legs, each exhale melts the forehead closer to the floor. Remembering to always lead with the heart and the forehead is secondary.

You may modify Toe Stretching Forward Fold by not coming into the forward fold and staying upright, or place a blanket under sitting bones, or squeeze all toes together in hands as oppose to interlacing fingers. Send each inhalation to awaken the entire foot, each exhalation casts out deep tension in the toes and arches.

The Lord guides our feet into many places throughout our life, spend time in this posture saying, "thank you" for Him always getting you to your destination, even if you have taken detours, praise Him for His constant and unconditional love that brings you back safely. Allow your detours to glorify Him.

SEATED POSTURES
GARLAND (MALASANA)

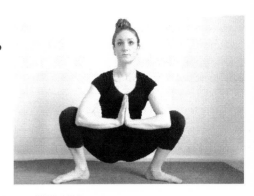

Getting into the Posture

1. Starting from a standing position, turn your toes outward and squat deeply, attempt to keep all four corners of the feet rooted to the earth.
2. Bring your palms to heart center as the elbows energetically press outward on the inner thighs, causing the torso to lengthen.
3. As hips gain flexibility, the heels will come closer together.

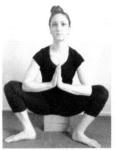
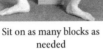
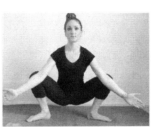
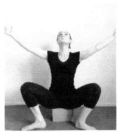

Sit on as many blocks as needed   Keep arms down   Lift arms high

Modification

- Sit on a chair, thighs parallel to earth, may need blocks underneath both feet, then fold the torso in between the thighs to your edge of the posture.
- Place a rolled blanket or mat underneath the heels. Eventually both feet, all four corners will connect with the earth.
- If you find the heels are very close to connecting to the ground, bring your feet closer together to assist in getting the entire foot rooted. Continue to breathe and allow the tailbone to reach down towards the ground.

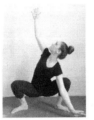
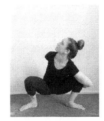
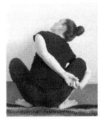

Reach and twist   Open shoulders with a bind   Blanket under heels

Deepen

- Opening up the arms, press the thighs outward.
- Hinging at the hips, forward fold the torso in between the legs. You can place the forearms on the ground, fingers pointing forward. Full expression of Garland Forward Fold is to externally rotate arms on the outside of thighs clasping the fingers or hands (may use a strap until achieved) near the small of the back. Soften the heels to the earth with each breath (You can also use a block to connect with the forehead in the full expression).
- Add a twist.
- Add a bind.

Use a blanket if needed for all modifications and deepening postures.

SEATED POSTURES
COW FACE (GOMUKHASANA)

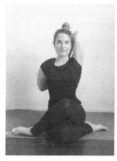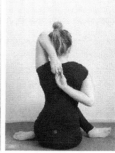

Getting into the Posture

1. From a Simple Seated or Double Pigeon pose, place one knee directly on top of the other. Both knees are bent.
2. Gently press each palm down on each ankle, stacking the knees directly in place.
3. Externally rotate the same arm, or opposite arm, as the top knee. Place palm on the thoracic region, palm facing inward, may also be the opposite arm as top leg.
4. The opposite arm internally rotates to reach for the fingers or strap if held in other palm.
5. Practice a Skull Draw by slightly tucking your chin in so that the back of your skull may touch the forearm, drishti or gaze, is straight out in front.

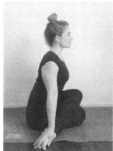 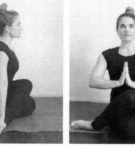 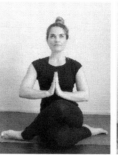 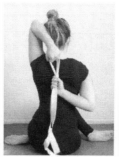 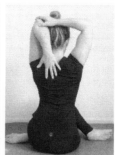

Practice lower body only   Hands to heart center   Use a strap   Practice only one side at a time

Modification

- Sit on a block or a rolled-up blanket.
- Stay upright, using no hand placement, and focus solely on the hip and knee joints.
- Bring your hands to heart center.
- Use a strap to connect your hands; inch your way to interlacing the fingers once the shoulders open.
- Assist your hand into the center of your back by pressing gently on the elbow.

Deepen

- If your fingers interlace, try moving both hands away (outward) from the torso.

To come into a deeper expression you may come into...

COW FACE FORWARD FOLD (GOMUKHA PASCHIMOTTANASANA)

Getting into the Posture

1. Keep your Cow Face pose active.
2. Hinge forward from the hip joints. (Cow face arms released in photo shown)
3. Press the top leg into the opposite thigh.
4. Keep a tight grip of the interlaced fingers so your back stays in alignment and your upper back muscles continue to strengthen.

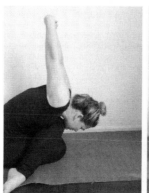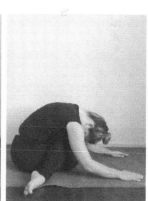

Breathe and surrender any self-doubt in this posture. Continue to inhale confidence in the Lord.

Modification

- Place the top foot on the ground so the knee is in the air to release some pressure.
- You may also fold using a strap for the hands, until eventually your shoulders and hips become open enough to come into full expression.
- Place block(s) under forehead.

Arms float forward   Simply rest arms

Whoever dwells in the shelter of the Most High will rest in the shadow of the Almighty. I will say of the Lord, "He is my refuge and my fortress, my God, in whom I trust. Psalm 91:1-2

SAGE FORWARD FOLD A (MARICHYASANA A)

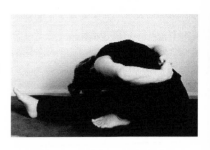

Getting into the Posture

1. From Staff Pose, bend one leg so the sole of the foot is planted on the earth.
2. On the same side as the bent leg, that arm extends up to lengthen the spine, torso then forward folds while the extended arms reaches to the inside of the bent inner thigh.
3. From the forward fold, the extended arm externally rotates around the outside edge of the bent thigh.
4. The opposite arm externally rotates clasping the other hands or fingers for a bind. Use a strap if needed.

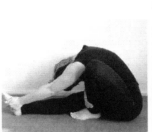 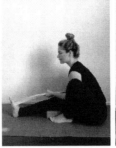 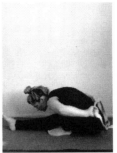

No bind   Use a strap and a block   Assisted bind with a strap

Modification

- Sit against a wall to assist with back support.
- Bring one knee up without forward folding.
- As you inhale, focus on lengthening the spine and increasing spinal muscles.
- Sit on a blanket for a more neutral pelvis, assisting in lower back and hip issues.
- Use a strap around the foot (the pad as opposed to the arch) and gently pull on the strap to focus more lengthening throughout the torso.
- Connect the hands into a bind to further open and stretch the shoulders.
- Keep your chin and heart lifted tall.

Deepen

- Close your eyes, "hug tightly" the leg muscles around the leg bones.
- Each exhalation brings you into a deeper forward fold and a deeper bind.
- Use a block to increase the extension of the reach and forward fold.
- Use a strap to bring your hands together behind you until your shoulders are flexible enough to complete the bind by clasping fingers or hands together.
- You may further deepen the posture by twisting the torso away from the bent knee.
- Relax your breath as you steady and anchor your heart and thoughts on Him.

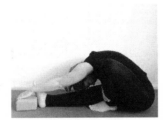

Forehead to knee and stretching
beyond the toes

I will meditate on Your precepts and regard Your ways. I shall delight in Your statutes;
I shall not forget Your word. Psalm 119:15-16

SAGE FORWARD FOLD B (MARICHYASANA B)

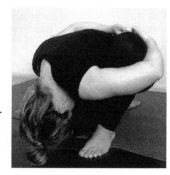

Getting into the Posture

1. From Staff Pose, tuck one leg underneath the buttock so the top of the foot is on earth and heel is connected to buttocks.
2. The same side as the bent leg, that arm extends up to lengthen the spine, torso then forward folds while the extended arm reaches to the inside of the bent inner thigh.
3. From the forward fold, the extended arm externally rotates around the outside edge of the bent thigh.
4. The opposite arm externally rotates clasping the other hand or fingers for a bind.

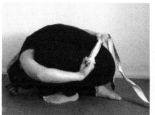 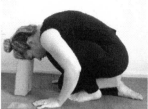

Strap to assist the bind   Block to assist the forehead and hips

Modification

- Sit against a wall to assist with back support.
- Bring one knee up without forward folding.
- Each inhale focuses on lengthening the spine and increasing spinal muscles.
- Use props to elevate tailbone and/or head.
- Sit on a blanket for a more neutral pelvis, assisting in lower back and hip issues.
- Keep one leg extended, and use a strap around the foot (the pad as opposed to the arch), then gently pull on strap to focus more on lengthening throughout the torso.
- You may also use a strap behind you. Focus on opening the shoulders to connect the hands into a bind.
- Keep your chin and heart lifted tall.

Deepen

- Close your eyes, "hug tightly" the leg muscles around the leg bones.
- Each exhalation brings you into a deeper forward fold and deeper bind.
- Continue to engage and "tuck yourself in."
- You may further deepen the posture by twisting your torso away from the bent knee.
- Practice Marichyasana C.
- In addition to the twist, opening up the shoulders, add a bind.

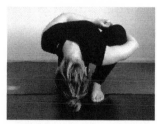 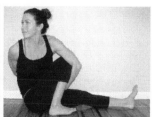

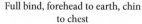

Full bind, forehead to earth, chin   Marichyasana C
to chest

Relax your breath as you steady and anchor your heart and thoughts. Exhalations release any trauma or tension, inhalations cleanse and renew. Surrender to being restored and awakened in every way here.

Prayer:
Lord, cleanse my heart and renew my mind.

HERO (VIRASANA)

Getting into the Posture

1. Bending both knees to place the shins on the earth, let the tailbone rest on the heels. For a gentler version, place a block in between legs.
2. Lengthen through your spine, as gravity pulls your tailbone down.
3. Your inner knees come together, as your feet separate hip width or beyond.
4. Depress the shoulder blades and lift the heart.

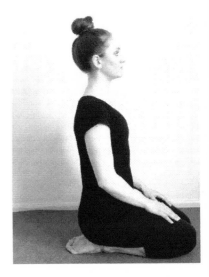

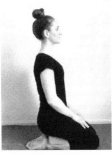 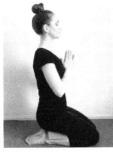

Modification

- Sit on a blanket, block, or bolster for a more neutral pelvis, assisting in lower back and hip issues.
- If you would like to forward fold, let a bolster hold your weight and enjoy a restorative Hero.

Sit on block   Close eyes, meditate

- Bring the toes together and sit on the heels. You may widen the knees if that is more comfortable.
- Place a blanket underneath the ankles, knees, and/or in between the knees and hamstrings.
- Settle into this posture.

Let each inhalation take in restoration. Every exhalation allows your heart to melt down and absorb healing.

Because Hero Pose reduces the blood supply to the legs, you may find this helps quiet your anxieties. Many people use Hero as a meditative posture for this reason. When you release the posture, enjoy the refreshing and invigorating fresh oxygen and blood flow to the body.

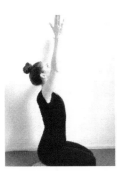

Deepen

- Clasp your fingers together and raise biceps towards your ears to lengthen your torso and spine.
- Clasp fingers at the small of your back expanding the chest and perhaps forward folding (not shown).
- Extend your arms high, keeping shoulders down, and lift the heart towards the sky.
- Take a deep forward fold.
- Rest your forehead on block or earth.
- Come into Reclining Hero.

Lift arms

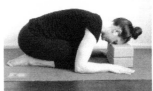 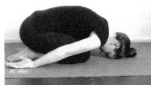

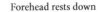

Forehead rests down   Blocks removed

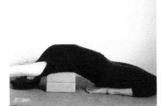 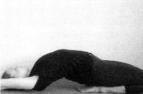 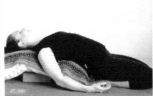 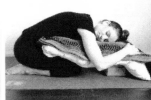

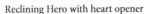

Reclining Hero with heart opener   Blocks removed   Restorative Reclining Hero   Restorative Forward Fold Hero

You do not always have to be strong. Without God, we can do nothing. Rest in His strength. He is strong; you are not. Lean on your hero, Christ. Rest in this truth here in this posture.

The Lord will march forth like a mighty hero; He will come out like a warrior, full of fury.
He will shout His battle cry and crush all His enemies. Isaiah 42:13

SEATED POSTURES
GATE (PARIGHASANA)

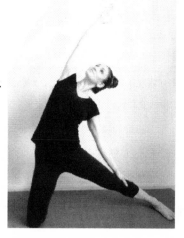

Getting into the Posture

1. Begin with both knees kneeling on the earth.
2. Extend one leg out to the side, pressing the foot into the earth. The bent leg remains, with knee directly under the hip for alignment.
3. Reach the opposite hand over towards the straight leg, palm down, opening up the entire side body.

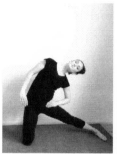 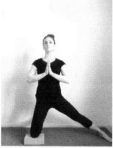 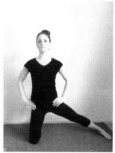 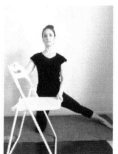

Decrease lateral flexion, no arms   Place a block under knee   Stay upright   Use a prop to assist

Modification

- Stay upright.
- Place a blanket or block under knee.
- If foot of the extended leg cannot connect with the ground, place a prop under the ball of foot or use a wall to press the foot into.
- Use the seat of a chair for assistance.
- Keep both arms on hips or by your side.
- Practice in a comfortable seated position, using blocks under forearms if needed.

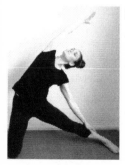

Deepen

- Deepen the side hinge.
- Each exhalation draws the lower hand closer to the foot of the extended leg.

Allow your exhalations to open the side body and release all worries, fear, doubts, and anxiety in this pose. Everything releases in this posture.

SEATED POSTURES
HERON (KROUNCHASANA)

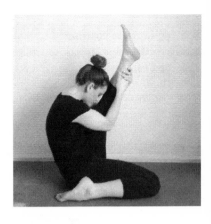

Getting into the Posture

1. From Staff Pose, bend one knee. Place your foot on the outside of your thigh, much like Hero but the foot is on the exterior and is connected to the thigh.
2. Straighten the opposite leg while bringing it upward towards your heart center. Use a strap in the beginning if necessary.
3. Keep the spine long and the torso straight.
4. The same side as the straightened leg, extend the same arm reaching around the exterior of the foot.
5. The opposite arm reaches for the opposite hand around the foot.

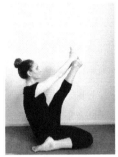 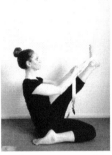 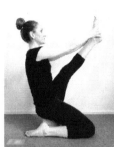 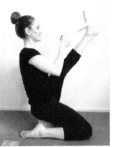

Leg does not come to torso

Place a strap around the foot

Elevate the tailbone

Practice with blocks and straps

Modification

- You may choose to remain in Head to Knee, keeping the extended leg on the ground.
- Bring leg as high as you can, forehead not coming to shin/knee.
- You can place a blanket or pillow under the sacrum, under the knee of the extended leg, and/or under the back foot (rests between the top of foot and floor).
- Clasp for the bottom of your foot; keep the knee bent in midair instead of extending the leg high.
- Use a strap around the raised leg.

Deepen

- Lead with your heart instead of the forehead, eventually connecting the shin of the extended leg to the forehead. When you lead with your heart, this keeps your spine straight so your torso does not cave in.
- Flex the toes towards heart center and widen or narrow your elbows with each breath.
- Place a block at the soles of extended leg's foot; wrap hands further around the block to deepen stretch.

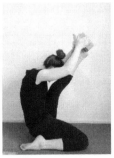 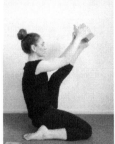

Head to knee, thigh to torso

Place a block to increase stretch

Inhalations bring in surrender, humility, vulnerability, and trust. Exhalations sweep your heart and spirit clean of anything else but these things. "Father, I breathe you into every fiber of my being. Draw me close to you."

SEATED POSTURES
LION (SIMHASANA)

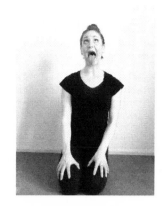

Getting into the Posture

1. From Hero pose, cross one ankle over the other behind you, and rest your tailbone on the top heel.
2. Actively spread out all ten fingers and press the palms on top of your thighs or knees.
3. Close your eyes.
4. Open your mouth as wide as you can, while taking a deep inhalation through the nose.
5. Stick out your tongue as far it can extend towards the chin.
6. As you exhale, open up your eyes as wide as you can, and look at the end of the nose, or upward.
7. On the next exhalation, perhaps try to gaze upward.
8. Switch crossed ankles and repeat same amount of breaths on the other side.

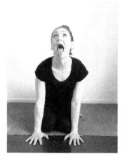

Come onto the palms

Modification

- Sit on a blanket, block, or bolster for a more neutral pelvis, assisting in lower back and hip issues.
- Stay in Hero Pose or do Lion's Face in Simple Seated Pose. Coming onto your hands will relieve some pressure in the feet and ankles.
- Bring your toes together and sit on the heels. You may widen the knees if that is more comfortable.
- Place a blanket under your ankles, knees, and/or between the knees and hamstrings.

Deepen

- Cross your legs so opposite heel is connecting with buttock.
- With each exhale, the jaw opens up a bit wider, the tongue extends a bit further, the eyes open a bit wider, and the exhalation goes from a forceful exhale to a loud sigh.
- You can practice in other postures as well. Try a forward fold or a Half Lotus Forward Fold, Cow Face, or Corpse Pose.

When you release the posture, enjoy the refreshing and invigorating fresh oxygen and blood flow to the body. Sit quietly in a comfortable seated position, close your eyes. Take inventory of what you are feeling. Make sure to relax your jaw and tongue. Do not clench the teeth and reverse the effects of what you just practiced.

Your inhalation reminds you to breathe in positive and edifying words. Your exhalations release negativity and words that no longer serve you.

The tongue can bring death or life; those who love to talk will reap the consequences.
Proverbs 18:21 New Living Translation

Always choose life and edification. Encourage others, and build them up. If what you are thinking about saying is not life, do not speak it.

ONE-LEGGED KING PIGEON (EKA PADA RAJAKAPOTASANA)

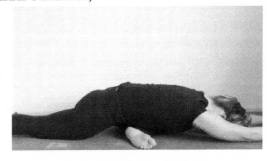

Getting into the Posture

1. From either a Table Top or Downward Facing Dog position, bring one knee near the same side wrist.
2. Slide the opposite leg back, so that it extends straight towards the back and not out to either side. The top of the foot remains on earth.
3. Lengthen through the torso as you lift your heart center upward, before walking your hands down.
4. Tailbone energetically lengthens downward, while the top of the crown reaches in the opposite direction.

Modification

- Stay upright, using as many props as needed for assistance.
- Place a blanket or similar prop under the bent leg's hip to neutralize hips and pelvis, assisting primarily with lower back and hip issues.
- If you would like to forward fold, let a bolster hold the weight of your torso, and enjoy a more Restorative Pigeon.
- Place a block (choose the best height) under the forehead.
- Place a block under each hand and stay tall.
- Inhalations focus on lengthening the top of the crown towards the sky and keeping the spine long as you root down into the blocks.
- Bend the back leg and use a strap with the back ankle.
- Use as many props as necessary in any posture.

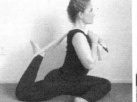

Prop underneath hip, block on forehead

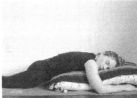

Stay upright with desired props

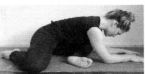

Modify the back leg and torso to desired depth

You may also come to a Reclining Pigeon. Lying on your back (supine), cross one ankle above the opposite knee, keep your sacrum and every vertebrae rooted to the earth. Place the foot that is resting on the thigh as far or near the opposite hip socket that is allowing a stretch in the hips. Staying center, breathe into the hips. Then you may rock side to side if you wish.

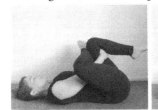

Clasp behind the knee

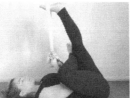

Place a strap around an extended leg

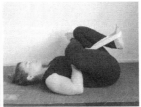

Place a strap around a bent leg

Stay upright and use a strap

Practice a Restorative Pigeon

Most of your tension, perhaps even the experience of a traumatic incident, lie in your hips, core, and center. Allow yourself time to release tension and trauma in whatever Pigeon you choose. Settling into your Pigeon, your exhalations expel clutter and debris, and your inhalations breathe in restoration and renewal.

Create in me a pure heart, Oh God, and renew a steadfast spirit within me. Psalm 51:10

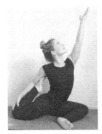

Tuck the foot into the armpit and reach upward

Deepen

- Come into (full) Pigeon after warming up with One-Legged Pigeon.
- Bending the back leg, bring the foot as close to the top of the head as possible.
- You may extend the opposite arm high. (shown)
- Bring the front foot away from the hip socket.
- Externally rotate both hands to clasp for the back foot or big toe.
- Use a strap around the ankle if needed.

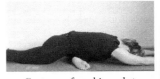

Foot away from hip socket

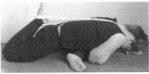

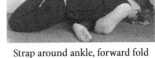

Strap around ankle, forward fold

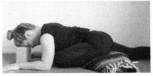

Bring hand to heart center, gaze upward

It is easy to hold your breath in back bends, but make sure to breathe. It's important to use your breath to work with your movements and postures. Make sure you give equal time on the other side.

In full expression of Pigeon as described here, continue to open and lift your heart to all possibilities with Christ. Let go of expectations and let your Pigeon soar.

SEATED POSTURES
SPLITS / MONKEY POSE (HANUMANASANA)

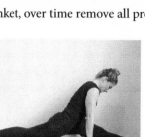

Getting into the Posture
1. From a Low Lunge, keep your hands on the earth or both hands firmly rooted to blocks as your front foot begins to inch its way towards the top of your mat.
2. Allow the hips to open and soften at your deepest expression of the splits.
3. You may also use a block under the groin area to rest down on.

Modification
- Use as many props and tools as you need in any posture. In your splits, you may use several props to assist you.
- Stay in a Low Lunge or a modified Crescent Pose.
- Use blocks under each hand. Start at the tallest height, then flat. When hips open up eventually, you can eliminate the blocks.
- Use a block under the tailbone, and rest down on it. Eventually switch the block to a blanket, over time remove all props and connect with the earth.

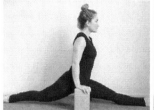 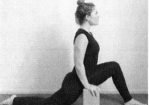 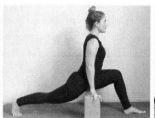

Use blocks to elevate the floor to you   Stay in low lunge with blocks   High lunge with blocks   Open hips, sit on as many blocks as needed

Deepen
- Forward fold, drawing the heart near the leg, forehead is secondary to heart leading. Reach for, or beyond the feet.
- Clasp opposite wrist or use a block at the sole of feet to reach beyond.
- Raise arms, extending and lengthening throughout the back of the arms towards the sky. Continue to reach the fingers up while drawing the rib cage down.
- Press into the earth with the back leg and energetically lift the back hamstring and front quadriceps up towards the sky.

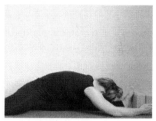

Forward fold with blocks at the end of foot to desired reach

Use your breath. Your inhalations lengthen your spine and with each exhalation, you are trusting more and releasing your fears. Release any doubts and know that you are exactly where you are supposed to be. Everything you have gone through has been for a reason and here you are, in this space, this incredible life-giving posture, inhaling the truth that you are exactly where you need to be. Let your bones absorb this truth.

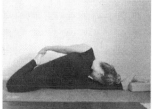 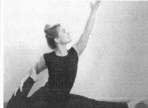 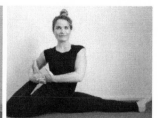

Clasp the back ankle, forward fold, reach beyond toes   Tuck the foot reach upward, breathe, reach   Clasp ankle and fingers

Consider it all joy, my brethren, when you encounter various trials, knowing that the testing of your faith produces endurance. And let endurance have its perfect result, so that you may be perfect and complete, lacking in nothing. But if any of you lacks wisdom, let him ask of God, who gives to all generously and without reproach, and it will be given to him. But he must ask in faith without any doubting, for the one who doubts is like the surf of the sea, driven and tossed by the wind. For that man ought not to expect that he will receive anything from the Lord, being a double-minded man, unstable in all his ways. James 1:2-5

SEATED POSTURES
SEATED LEG BEHIND THE HEAD (EKA PADA SIRSASANA)

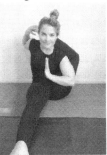

Getting into the Posture

1. From Staff Pose, come into Cradle. Bring your foot into opposite crease of the elbow; interlace all ten fingers as you hold the leg, as if you are rocking a baby. This will open up your hips and prepare you more for the pose.
2. Releasing Cradle, tuck your shoulder under the knee that was in Cradle.
3. Be sure to sit as tall as you can throughout this posture.
4. Place your foot behind your neck, then hook or lock it into place.
5. Open your heart in this posture; place your palms at heart center.
6. Keep your breath steady and calm.

Modification

- Stay in Cradle, opening up the hips while holding onto the foot.
- Do not come into full expression. Gradually work up to placing the leg behind your head without concaving inward.

If you cannot place your leg behind your head while your neck and shoulders alone support the leg, you are not ready to place the leg behind you. It is important that once you rest the leg behind you, you are able to lift your collarbone and heart towards the sky for proper alignment, without the back leg falling off.

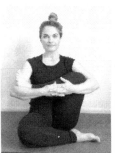
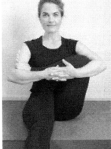
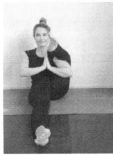
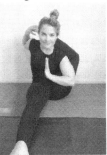

| Cradle with bent leg | Cradle with leg extended | Place leg on arm only | Hold foot |

Deepen

- Externally rotate the hip joint and anchor the thigh behind your arm.
- Allow your upper back, shoulders and neck to support the leg, while your strong core, heart and chest expand and lift towards the sky.
- Breathe.

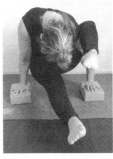
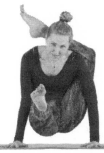

- Further deepen this posture by creating an arm balance.
- Bring extended leg off the ground and connect the forehead and chin to the leg.
- Further deepen this posture by forward folding with leg anchored behind you, hand to ground, heart center or bind.
- Make sure to repeat on the other side for the same amount of time.

Add desired arm balance

Remember the hips are where most of your tension lies; perhaps even a traumatic incident is trapped there. Allow yourself time and patience in this posture. Settling into your Leg Behind the Head, no expectations, just breathing, relaxing and allowing your hips patience and ease.

Embrace your journey. Your exhalations expel impatience and frustration, while your inhalations breathe in time.

Wash me, and I will be whiter than snow. Let me hear joy and gladness; let the bones you have crushed rejoice. Hide your face from my sins and blot out all my iniquity. Create in me a pure heart, Oh God, and renew a steadfast spirit within me. Do not cast me from your presence or take your Holy Spirit from me. Restore to me the joy of your salvation and grant me a willing spirit, to sustain me. Psalm 51:7-12

Prayer:
Heavenly Father, please help me to create space and time for You. Help me to be still. I no longer want to rush around believing that I do not have time for You. Today, I reaffirm that You are the most important thing in my life and that my life cannot function without You. I must hear from You. I will look forward to our daily appointment together, on or off my mat. Thank You for being my everything at all times.
Amen.

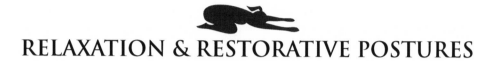

RELAXATION & RESTORATIVE POSTURES

For I will restore health to you, and your wounds I will heal, declares the Lord. Jeremiah 30:17

RELAXATION & RESTORATIVE POSTURES

God has told His people, "Here is a place of rest; let the weary rest here.
This is a place of quiet rest." Isaiah 28:12

The Bible tells us repeatedly to be still. God often repeats Himself throughout the Bible. I believe it is because it touches on a subject that we need to pay close attention to. So often, He tells us to "sit, rest, be still and trust." He must be trying to get His point across as He commands us so often to do these things.

Relaxation postures are the perfect way to quiet our hearts and minds and turn them toward God. In the Bible, meditation means "mumbling scripture." We can dwell on His Word and all the good reports in any relaxing and restorative pose. Meditation also means to deeply ponder or contemplate. So while resting and being restored, we can contemplate, deeply ponder and chew on His word.

There are no complicated postures in relaxation or restorative poses. Most of these postures are done with props such as straps, blocks, blankets, bolsters and eye pillows. Restorative postures release deep tension throughout the body, but specifically in the ligaments and tendons. These postures can draw you closer to the Lord as you become still and quiet. This could become your favorite way to spend time with Him. The more you practice relaxation postures, the better you will become at finding stillness. For many, this may prove to be the most challenging asana family of them all, because it requires pausing, withdrawing, slowing down and becoming still.

The posture of our prayers, as well as our prayers themselves, say much about our relationship with God. Lying on your back is a humbled, vulnerable and surrendered position. God loves it when we humble ourselves and surrender to Him. These are the times He is able to speak directly into our spirit from His spirit! Relax, listen, surrender and be restored!

For this reason the Father loves me, because I lay down my life so that I may take it again. No one has taken it away from me, but I lay it
down on my own initiative. I have authority to lay it down, and I have authority to take it up again.
This commandment I received from my Father. John 10:17-18

First, I want to declare that God can restore you beyond the "original state." He can, and He will.

Is something in your life broken? Has the enemy stolen something or someone from you? Do you cringe when an enemy who attacked you gets blessed? Are there times when it seems as though the wicked and corrupt are the only blessed people? There is great news for you and me.

Zechariah 9:12 *promises* this,
Return to the stronghold, oh prisoners who have the hope; this very day I am declaring that I will restore double to you.

This is from the American Standard Version and I love it because it says return. As a child of the most high God, the only way we can be restored is to first return. Throughout scripture, we are the ones who must knock first, seek first and come to Him first. Then He opens the door and we are found and *then* He comes to us. We must first return.

The following relaxation postures are a perfect way to return to God. Do these postures in a quiet place, with no distractions. You will find yourself looking forward to this time with your Maker. As with other appointments you set, it may be necessary to set an appointment for this time with God.

Try not to let anything or anyone stop you from getting still before the Lord each day. There is an enemy and he would like nothing more than to keep you from doing the will of God and sharing Christ with others. God is so good. He longs and waits to spend time with us, no matter what we have done or how far away we have gotten from Him. It does not matter where we have been or what we have done; God is a good God and He has good plans for us. *We can always return to Him.* You may have fallen so far away from Him. Or perhaps the enemy is constantly chirping in your ear that you could never be in God's good graces because of what you have done or who you are. The devil is a liar! Do not believe him for one more second. There is always forgiveness, mercy and grace with the Lord. His unconditional love never fails and He has promised to never forsake you (Hebrews 13:5).

Therefore all who devour you will be devoured; and all your adversaries, every one of them, will go into captivity; and those who plunder
you will be for plunder, and all who prey upon you I will give for prey. For I will restore you to health and I will heal you of your wounds,
declares the Lord Because they have called you an outcast, saying: "It is Zion; no one cares for her." Jeremiah 30:16-17

Here, Jeremiah wrote about the restoration of Judah and Israel after extravagant worship of false idols and gods. He compares Judah to a prostitute, as the nation had completely abandoned God after the righteous King Josiah died. Yet, God promised He would restore their health and heal their wounds. Grace is not fair, is it? It is *unmerited favor.* Friend, this is great news. Because if we all got what we deserved, we would all be up a creek! We think to ourselves, "But they don't deserve all that goodness. It's not fair." *None* of us deserve His unconditional love and forgiveness but He gives it to us every day, free. That is great grace! He bestows upon us grace piled upon grace!

RELAXATION & RESTORATIVE POSTURES

I will come to you and fulfill my gracious promise to bring you back to this place. For I know the plans I have for you, declares the Lord, plans to prosper you and not to harm you, plans to give you hope and a future. Jeremiah 29:10-11

Any time you feel lost, weak or broken, practice your restorative postures and meditate upon what Jeremiah declared about your Heavenly Father. Rest in His grace: your *unmerited favor.*

Relaxation and restorative postures are important to take time *in*, as they integrate the effects of your practice as a whole. Most important, these postures are vital as a time for listening *to* the Lord. We do not always have to come to Him with a list of things we want from Him. We can be with our Father in sweet simplicity without saying a word. This is, after all, a time to be renewed and restored. Allow these postures to let Him captivate you while you are still. Absorb His calming, healing and restoring to wholly take over you. This is what a restorative practice can do: calm your anxious thoughts and heal your deep wounds and broken heart. These postures will also rejuvenate and energize your entire body.

Relaxation poses are perfect for meditating on all His promises. If you practice these postures during a series of postures or in a sequence, they can be the most difficult postures of your practice. It isn't always easy to be still, yet conscious. These postures are typically done at the end of practice, as well as incorporated throughout a sequence of postures. Child's pose, for instance, is a restorative posture that many use to take a break from a series or to let the body simply absorb your physical activity. Corpse Pose, or Resting Angel, has been called the "most favorite" and the "most difficult" posture. It may be both of these for you. Resting Angel is lying on your back, usually at the end of practice, and if so, the eyes close and face relaxes. This should be how you end every practice. It will allow your body, bones, muscles, mind, spirit, and all your systems to absorb and receive the blessing of that day's practice. *Ah, absorb.*

If you are practicing restorative postures without a sequence, spend as much time in them as you need. Perhaps placing an eye pillow over the eyes and resting will be necessary at times. It is a time of stillness, calm and peace with the Lord. This will be a safe place where you can be lulled to sleep and rest with your Father. Again, in restorative yoga, there are no complicated poses or tensions placed on the body and props are typically used in all the postures. Your quiet space should include anything you choose to assist you in restorative poses (A pillow or bolster, blocks, chair, blanket, eye pillow, etc.). For example, you can rest your legs on the seat of a chair. A blanket softens the sacrum to the floor. A pillow is under the head and an eye pillow over the eyes.

Resting Angel is a deeply restorative pose and by far the most important posture of your practice. It will allow your body to realign, restore and absorb everything you practice. The more you practice relaxation postures the better you will become at finding stillness, surrendering your "stuff," and hearing from God. These poses can release deep tension, not just physically, but in the mind, spirit and emotional heart as well.

Speak tenderly to Jerusalem, and proclaim to her that her hard service has been completed, that her sin has been paid for, that she has received from the Lord's hand double for all her trouble. Isaiah 40:2

You may need to read that again. Your *hard service has been completed!*

Benefits of restorative postures include, but are not limited to:

- Awakens the legs, alleviates, or is therapeutic for varicose veins and other circulatory issues.
- Relieves the heart of any stressful duties (if one has high blood pressure or heart disease for example), as well as improves circulation.
- Gently stretches the hips, thighs and ankles.
- Relieves neck and back pain when head is supported.
- Improves digestion, circulation and respiratory systems.
- Therapeutic for headaches, migraines, backache, sciatica, menstruation and menopause discomfort, infertility, insomnia, arthritis, osteoporosis, sinusitis, vertigo and glaucoma.
- Improves concentration and mental focus.
- Relieves depression, stress and anxiety.
- Relieves mental and physical exhaustion.
- Calming and centering.

Cautions include, but are not limited to:
- Serious knee, hip or back injury.
- Back, neck or shoulder injury.
- Pregnant women should use modifications and avoid deep forward folds during second or third trimester.

DIG INTO THE WORD. YOUR SOUL WORK; HEBREWS 4
A MEDITATION FOR RESTORATIVE POSTURES

THE POSTURES

LEGS UP THE WALL (VIPARITA KARANI)

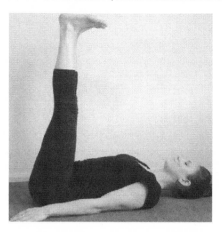

Getting into the Posture

1. Lie on your back, then use a wall, or simply extend your legs towards the sky.
2. Keep your spine long and skull on the ground.
3. Relax your feet for a restorative Legs up the Wall, or engage the legs by pressing your heels up towards the sky.
4. Use a blanket under the sacrum if desired.

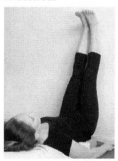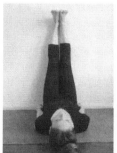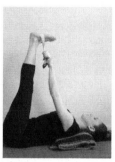

Place legs on a wall, use as many props as desired

Modification

- Use a blanket under the shoulders and pelvis.
- Keep your tailbone close to the wall; use blocks and/or blanket.
- Practice with a strap and blanket(s).
- Place your legs on a wall; use as many props as desired.

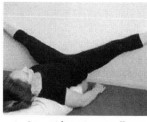

Legs wide against a wall
(or no wall)

Deepen

- Open legs wide.
- Use a block underneath the shoulder blades to open the heart center.

Counter Poses

- Fish
- Resting Angel
- Lie on Belly

CHILD'S POSE (BALASANA)

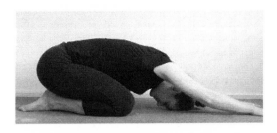

Come, let us worship and bow down, let us kneel before the Lord our Maker, for He is our God, and we are the people of His pasture and the sheep of His hand. Today, if you would hear His voice. Psalm 95:6-7

Getting into the Posture

1. Kneeling with the tops of the feet on the earth, bring your big toes to touch.
2. Separate the knees out wide (if desired) as you fold your torso to rest between the thighs.
3. Place your hands to your sides, or outstretch arms above your head, palms facing up and rest the forehead down to the earth or onto a block.
4. Rest in this posture, or practice Child's Pose during a sequence for rest.

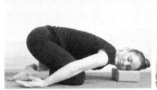
Block between thighs and under cheek

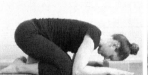
Block between thighs forehead rests on block

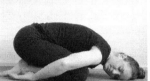
Head rests down

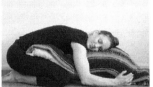
Blocks under bolster or pillow, torso rests

Modification:

- Use a rolled up blanket or block between back of thighs and your calves.
- Place a block/blanket under forehead.
- Place a bolster or pillow under torso.
- Use as many props as needed.
- Practice Table Top on all fours.

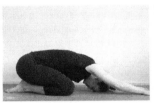
Stretch fingertips as far as you can while sinking hips back and downward

Deepen

- Walk hands out, roll shoulder blades down back.
- Roll the eyebrow bone and forehead from side to side.
- Open knees wide with outstretched arms.
- Stretch fingertips as far as you can while sinking hips back and downward.

To further deepen, practice...

PUPPY / EXTENDED CHILD'S POSE and THREAD THE NEEDLE

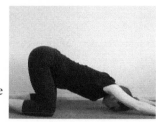

Getting into the Posture
1. From Child's Pose, come to a Table Top position.
2. Slowly lower your torso down towards the ground by extending or walking your hands in front of you. You may place your forehead on the ground or your chin on the mat, if your neck allows.
3. Continue to reach your fingers forward opening up shoulders and armpits. Keep the hips directly above the knees as your heart is pulled energetically towards the earth.

Puppy or Extended Child's Pose

THREAD THE NEEDLE

Getting into the Posture
1. From Extended Child's Pose, place one arm under the other.
2. Rest the cheek on the ground, or look the opposite way to stretch the throat and neck.

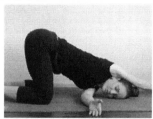 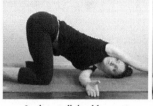 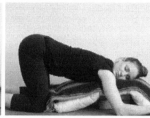

Neutral neck   Look up, roll shoulder open   Rest

Thread the Needle Variation in Puppy Dog Pose; although not comfortable, looking the opposite way of the bottom arm to stretch the throat and neck, this will stimulate the nervous, respiratory and circulatory systems greatly. It could also be therapeutic for asthma depending on the severity.

I am the Lord, and I will bring you out from under the yoke of the Egyptians. I will free you from being slaves to them, and I will redeem you with an outstretched arm. Exodus 6:6

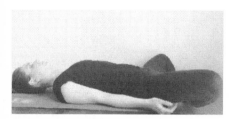

RECLINING BOUND ANGLE (SUPTA BADDHA KONASANA)

God has told His people, "Here is a place of rest; let the weary rest here. This is a place of quiet rest."
Isaiah 28:12

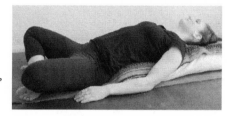

Getting into the Posture
1. From Bound Angle, slowly walk your elbows behind you as you come onto your back.
2. Use props as described below.
3. Allow gravity to pull the knees down so the hips and groins open up to release tension.

Modification
- Lifting the feet onto a block, choose the best height that suits the flexibility of your hips (The tallest height will be the most intense).
- Place a block or blanket under the head, neck, and/or sacrum.
- Incorporate several modifications and come into a restorative Reclining Bound Angle.
- Use a blanket or bolster that supports the entire spine and head.
- Place blankets under each outer thigh.
- A strap around the ankles and hips will provide additional support, as well as an eye pillow placed over the eyes for a restorative Reclining Bound Angle.

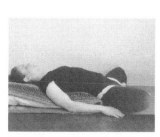

Restorative Reclining Bound Angle

Deepen
- Place a block at desired height between your shoulder blades, allowing a heart opener and chest expansion within the posture.
- Bring the strap, or the feet, closer to the groin as your hips gain flexibility.
- Place a block under the sacrum.

DIG INTO THE WORD. YOUR SOUL WORK; PSALM 139
A MEDITATION FOR RECLINING BOUND ANGLE

As you practice Reclining Bound Angle and other similar meditative postures, remember He knows your most inward thoughts. He created you, and you are fearfully and wonderfully made! Do not let the enemy, or anyone/anything the enemy would try to use, tell you anything else. God's plans are for you to prosper and be in good health, just as your soul prospers. Check in with your soul during this time of meditation. Ask yourself, "How is it with my soul today?"

Dear friend, I pray that you may enjoy good health and that all may go well with you, even as your soul is getting along well. 3 John 1:2

RECLINING BIG TOE (SUPTA PADANGUSTHASANA)

Getting into the Posture

1. Lying on your back, bring one leg up towards the head and grab for the big toe.
Option: Grab for the ankle or calf, use a strap around the foot.
2. Bend the resting leg if you have lower back issues, or keep it extended.

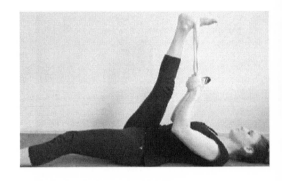

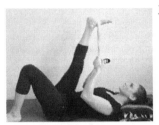

Modification

- Place a blanket under sacrum and/or neck.
- Bend resting leg so the sole of the foot is on ground to protect your lumbar region.
- Use a strap, bend lower leg and blanket as a pillow.

Use a strap, bend lower leg and blanket as a pillow

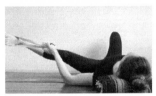

Deepen

- Open leg up to same side.
- You can also gaze opposite direction.
- With the opposite hand, reach around the head to clasp for the strap or the opposite foot; this includes a beautiful side body stretch.
- Hold for a minute before switching sides.

Open leg to the side

RECLINING PIGEON (SUPTA EKA PADA RAJAKAPOTASANA)

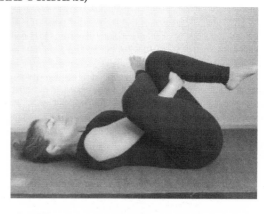

Getting into the Posture

1. Lying on your back, bending both knees so the soles of the feet are on the ground, cross one ankle just above the kneecap of the opposite leg.
2. You may keep the sole of your foot on the ground, or lift the foot up to bring the knee into the heart center.
3. Clasp hands behind the hamstring if possible, while keeping the sacrum rooted to the earth.
4. Practice a skull draw, which is slightly tucking the chin down towards the chest, creating a long spine.
5. Gaze is directly upward or rest the eyes.
6. Release and switch.

Modification

- Place a blanket under your sacrum and/or neck.
- Bend resting leg so the sole of the foot is on ground to protect lumbar region.
- Use a strap on the sole of the bottom foot.

Deepen

- Hold for a several minutes before switching sides.
- Extend the non-crossed leg upward, may also use a strap around the sole of the extended foot.
- Keeping pigeon legs, come into a spinal twist, releasing the sole of the crossed leg on to the ground while the other leg rests completely down. May also look the opposite direction of the legs.
- Gently rock from side to side.

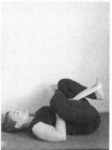 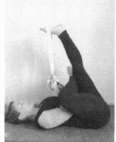

Practice using strap   Extended leg with strap

RECLINING HERO (SUPTA VIRASANA)

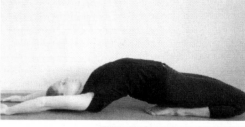

Getting into the Posture

1. From Seated Hero, slowly walk your elbows behind you as you come onto your back.
2. Use props if needed as described in modifications.
3. Bring knees back together if they have come apart, and gently roll your knees inward towards one another.

Modification

- Stay in Seated Hero.
- Place a block or blanket underneath the sacrum and/or head.
- Use a blanket or bolster that supports the entire spine and head, consider an eye pillow.
- Rest on the elbows or use blocks that are placed behind the hips to rest hands on, as opposed to coming down entirely on the back.
- Lay on one side and bring the ankle near the buttock.
- Use a strap if necessary and repeat on the other side.
- Use as many props as needed.
- Focus on the quadriceps stretching on each side as you practice one side at a time.
- As you gain flexibility in your thighs, try the full version of Reclining Hero.

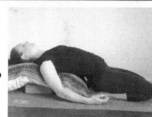

Use as many props as needed

Deepen

- Place a block at desired height between the shoulder blades, allowing a heart opener and chest expansion within the posture.
- Raise your palms up toward the ceiling, perpendicular to the floor and gently rock from side to side.
- Raise hands behind your head; place the back of the hand on the floor so the palm faces up as you open the armpits and shoulders.
- Raise hands behind your head as you place the forearms on the ground, grabbing for opposite elbows.

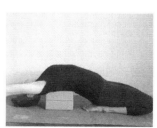

Blocks with outstretched arms

CORPSE / RESTING ANGEL POSE (SAVASANA)

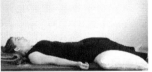

Getting into the Posture

1. Lying on your back, spread all limbs out so nothing is bent or constricted.
2. Let your feet splay open and your palms lay natural.
3. Close your eyes, focus on the breath and do not let the mind wander or worry. Still your thoughts on the Lord. Meditate on His promises and consider what He has brought you through.
4. Use as many props as needed, including an eye pillow, maybe lavender scented to increase relaxation.
5. Explore a narrow stance or spread limbs wide like a large star and simply feel the differences.

Modification

- Place a blanket under the sacrum, between the shoulder blades, and/or head.
- Bend both legs so the soles of the feet are on the ground to protect your lumbar region.
- Use a bolster to place under the knees.
- Use a chair to alleviate any pressure.
- Place a prop between legs to keep hips in alignment.
- If you are pregnant, especially if you're in your second and third trimester, lay on your side with a pillow or bolster between your thighs.
- Use the seat of a chair and block or pillow.
- Place a bolster under knees, block under neck.
- Use a blanket for a pillow and neck support.

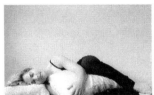
Place prop between legs to keep hips in alignment

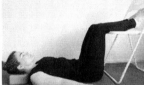
Use the seat of a chair and block or pillow

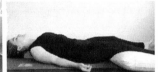
Place bolster under knees, block under neck

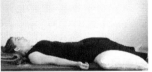
Use a blanket for a pillow and neck support

Deepen

- Focus on quieting your mind and simply being still.

Counter Pose

- Corpse/Resting Angel Pose should conclude your practice or for resting during a (any) sequence of asanas.
- If Resting Angel Pose is practiced as a rest in between postures, you may wish to practice Wind Relieving Pose, Bridge, Wheel or any inversion if you want continued energy after your practice.
- If it concludes your practice, use a blanket, blocks, eye pillow, aromatherapy and whatever else will help relieve tension and stress.

DIG INTO THE WORD. YOUR SOUL WORK; PSALM 46
A MEDITATION FOR RESTING ANGEL

Do not cast me away from Your presence and do not take Your Holy Spirit from me. Restore to me the joy of Your salvation and sustain me with a willing spirit. Then I will teach transgressors Your ways, and sinners will be converted to You. Psalm 51:11-13

Prayer:

Dear Heavenly Father, I come before You and surrender all my anxious thoughts and busy, needless worries. I ask that Your Spirit continually remind me today to be still and help quiet my heart. I know that You have things You need to tell me. Today I pray that I may be able to hear these things. I want to know You more. I pray that You reveal Your hidden mysteries and treasures to me today and that You would enlighten the eyes of my understanding. Thank you Father that I never have to worry, doubt, or fear. Today I rest in You. Today I trust in Your promises. In your precious, sweet, and mighty name, Amen!

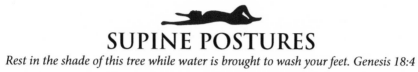

SUPINE POSTURES

Rest in the shade of this tree while water is brought to wash your feet. Genesis 18:4

I am the good shepherd, and know my sheep, and am known of mine. As the Father knows me, even so know I the Father: and I lay down my life for the sheep. And other sheep I have, which are not of this fold: them also I must bring, and they shall hear my voice; and there shall be one fold, and one shepherd. John 10:14-16

Sometimes in life, we just have to come to the Father and lay it all down. We need to cast all our cares and heavy burdens upon Him, and let go of the things that we try to carry ourselves.

The wonderful thing about combining our faith with yoga, is we can come to our mat and be still. We create this amazingly intimate space to worship with our whole self, to lay down and quiet our hearts and minds. I have learned that the stillness and quietness actually leads me to His voice. John 10 says, "That His sheep know His voice." Too often, we allow the noise of life to drown out His voice. God doesn't yell at us, but He always speaks in a still, small voice. How would we ever hear this small voice if our world is so loud? When was the last time you simply listened?

During our study of the supine postures that have yet to be explored, find a posture that speaks to you personally. Come before God, lie down on your back, and turn your heart and eyes upon Him. Some of the following postures can be relaxing and restorative. Think of the song written by Helen H. Lemmel that says,

"Turn your eyes upon Jesus, look full in His wonderful face, and the things of earth will grow strangely dim, in the light of His glory and grace"

BE STILL

By this time, I hope you have realized the importance of rest, being still, and allowing God to work in the times of quietness and stillness. As we explored with restorative postures, supine postures, or on the back, will remind us again, to rest in His presence. If we do not create this time of rest, we cannot be restored, and therefore we cannot be revived to energy, health, and wholeness. Do you need to rest? Does your soul need to be quieted? What about your anxious thoughts and doubts? Worrying does not add one moment to your life; it actually deducts from your life, so stop worrying! Dear friend, it is time for you to rest, embrace, and allow yourself to find stillness, often.

Today we are bombarded with distractions and obstacles that vie for our attention. We exhaust ourselves to the point of walking around like zombies. Hopelessness and discouragement creep in, and if we are not careful, we can spiral downward fast. When we are exhausted, the enemy can come in like a flood. Our hopelessness and exhaustion leaves us defenseless in the face of our enemy. Do not become weary! How do we do that? We find rest and allow God to restore, revive, and cleanse our souls.

Rest in the shade of this tree while water is brought to wash your feet. Genesis 18:4

Does this verse speak to you as it does me? I picture a countryside with open meadows and a simple home on the land. I see a large willow tree, me, lying on my back, resting underneath its shade in the cool breeze. Then I imagine the Lord Himself, washing my feet. Just the simple thought of this scene brings me rest.

What about you? Are you tired? Do you long for such peace? Are you able to surrender, or lay down your distractions, noise, things to do, anxieties, fears, and doubts to allow the Lord to wash your feet? Will you allow the Lord to cleanse the muddy waters that can so easily overwhelm? I believe you want to do so. Perhaps you can take a few moments right now, turn your thoughts on Him, and rest in perfect peace.

And who of you by being worried can add a single hour to his life? And why are you worried about clothing? Observe how the lilies of the field grow; they do not toil nor do they spin, yet I say to you that not even Solomon in all his glory clothed himself like one of these. Matthew 6:27-29

Think about Luke 12:27; Imagine a beautiful lily trying to clothe itself and toil in its own strength to grow and bloom. The lily is nourished, lives, and thrives because it is rooted in the One who controls the elements. It grows, blossoms, and flourishes from an internal place. It does not fret or worry about how it will grow or survive.

What if we did the same? What if we relinquished *(voluntarily abandoned)* our worries of the day and truly enjoyed what the Lord blesses us with every day? Could you get used to this kind of peaceful living? Well friend, this is how we are supposed to live.

You keep him in perfect peace whose mind is stayed on You, because he trusts in You. Isaiah 26:3

SUPINE POSTURES

The Message version reads:

People with their minds set on You, You keep completely whole,
steady on their feet, because they keep at it and don't quit.
Isaiah 26:3

I don't know about you, but I desire to live and be whole. How do we do this? We set our minds on Him. We don't give up, get discouraged, weary or exhausted. We keep at it and do not quit! We stay in the Word and daily meditate on His promises to us.

A scripture you may be familiar with is Jeremiah 29:11,
For I know the plans that I have for you, declares the Lord, plans to prosper you and not to harm you.

Allow me to elaborate on the surrounding verses.

Make yourselves at home there and work for the country's welfare. "Pray for Babylon's well-being. If things go well for Babylon, things will go well for you." Yes, believe it or not, this is the Message from God-of-the-Angel-Armies, Israel's God: "Don't let all those so-called preachers and know-it-alls who are all over the place there take you in with their lies. Don't pay any attention to the fantasies they keep coming up with to please you. They're a bunch of liars preaching lies – and claiming I sent them! I never sent them, believe me." God's Decree: This is God's Word on the subject: "As soon as Babylon's seventy years are up and not a day before, I'll show up and take care of you as I promised and bring you back home. I know what I'm doing. I have it all planned out – plans to take care of you, not abandon you, plans to give you the future you hope for. "When you call on me, when you come and pray to me, I'll listen. When you come looking for me, you'll find me. I'll make sure you won't be disappointed." God's Decree. "I'll turn things around for you. I'll bring you back from all the countries into which I drove you" - God's Decree - "bring you home to the place from which I sent you off into exile. You can count on it. "But for right now, because you've taken up with these newfangled prophets who set themselves up as 'Babylonian specialists,' spreading the word 'God sent them just for us!' God is setting the record straight.
Jeremiah 29:7-16, The Message Version

It goes on to say how we don't have to worry about our enemies because God is taking care of them too. This is Jeremiah's letter to the captives in Babylon, telling them to be quiet there. He tells them to lay aside distractions, false prophets (those who say they are of God, but lie and deceive), and the noise of life. He tells us to enjoy what the Lord has brought us to and find peace and rest. I love *The Message Version* because it reads slightly different from all the other versions that say *"plans to take care of us and give us a future and a hope…"* The Message says, *"plans to give you the future you hope for."*

"Wait, what? The future I hope for?" you may ask. Yes! The future *you* hope for!

If we are Christ followers, then the future God hopes for us is [actually] the future we hope for ourselves, and vice versa. It is interchangeable. When we receive Him, we receive a new beginning and His will for our life. What matters to us matters to God, and what matters to God matters to us. His plans are to give you the future *you* hope for! This is the great exchange. So, what do you hope for? Have you written it down and made it clear? This vision should align completely with God's will because it is the future, the vision that He hopes for you and the future that you hope for. It is one in the same because we are one with Him.

Write the vision; make it plain on tablets, so that a herald may run with it. Habakkuk 2:2

Then rest. Rest in knowing that He has it all planned out.
"I know what I'm doing. I have it all planned out - plans to take care of you, not abandon you, plans to give_____ the future you hope for.
Your name here

Now that we know how important it is to rest and trust the Lord, let's explore more postures that are supine. These postures are the perfect way to rest, be revived, restored and simply to meditate on trusting the Lord.

SUPINE POSTURES

Supine postures can also be explored in twists, seated or inverted postures. Here, we will cover a few more supine postures that are not considered as restorative poses. As a reminder, supine postures are excellent for resting and restoring, but are also great for realigning the entire body, improving the circulation, digestion and respiratory systems, as well as improving concentration, focus, coordination and memory. More benefits include stress and tension release, increased flexibility, specifically in the hips and spine. They will also improve assimilation and elimination. Supine posture can stretch ligaments, muscles and nerves while strengthening, opening and relaxing the entire body.

The majority of these postures can be quite relaxing and gentle, which is great for those with limitations. You can modify and use props with many postures to assist in relaxing or deepening the pose. Those who suffer from major medical issues can enjoy supine postures for healing.

Pregnant women in their second or third trimester should use a cushion under buttocks and sacrum areas. Avoid extreme stretching and twisting during the third trimester.

Benefits of supine postures include but are not limited to:
- Improves alignment of the spine, improving posture.
- Improves circulation.
- Can relieve digestion, constipation, gastritis, menstrual and menopause symptoms.
- Therapeutic for mild sciatica, osteoporosis, tension backaches, glaucoma, vertigo and asthma.
- Therapeutic for practitioners with limitations such as pregnancy, trauma, AIDS, arthritis, cancer, diabetes, fibromyalgia, MS, PTSD, Down Syndrome and immobility.
- Relieves fatigue, anxiety and mild depression.
- Calming, centering and grounding yet revitalizes, awakens and restores.

Cautions include but are not limited to:
- Severe back, shoulder, wrist, knee or hip injury.
- Pregnancy (depending on trimester), diarrhea, hernia or ulcer.

DIG INTO THE WORD. YOUR SOUL WORK; JOHN 10:14-16
A MEDITATION FOR SUPINE POSTURES

I am the good shepherd, and I know my own and my own know me, even as the Father knows me and I know the Father; and I lay down my life for the sheep. I have other sheep, which are not of this fold; I must bring them also, and they will hear my voice; and they will become one flock with one shepherd. John 10:14-16

THE POSTURES

KNEES TO CHEST / WIND RELIEVING & HALF WIND RELIEVING / APANA (PAVANAMUKTASANA)

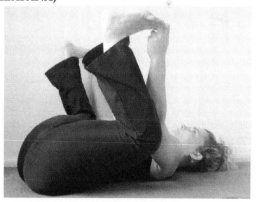

Getting into the Posture

1. Lying on your back, bring both knees to your chest.
2. Wrap your arms just below both knees.
3. Clasp for fingers, wrists, forearms or elbows.
4. If your head has come off the mat, make sure to lower it back down, creating a long spine.
5. As you inhale, feel your belly rise against your thighs; lengthen your arms and slightly draw your chin into your chest (Chin to chest is also known as skull draw; it creates the longest spine possible).
6. As you exhale, engage your arms as you bring your knees into your heart center. Imagine the knees pressing the toxins out of your body.
7. Energetically press your knees with your elbows. Be sure to press the sacrum into the earth, as opposed to lifting it up on the exhalations.
8. Repeat for as long as needed.

Modification

- Place a blanket under your sacrum and/or neck.
- Use a strap at the bottom of your feet.
- Bring your knees to the outside your torso, and practice this version for second and third trimester of pregnancy.
- Practice Half Wind Relieving Pose (Ardha Pavanamuktasana).

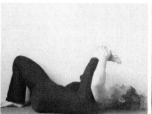
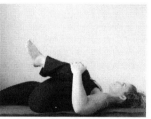

Bring knees to outside of torso   Practice one leg at a time

Deepen

- Use in a flow with Bridge, Wheel or Shoulder Stand.

HAPPY BABY / JOYFUL BABY (ANANDA BALASANA)

Getting into the Posture

1. Lying on your back, bring both knees in toward the chest.
2. Keep your tailbone on the earth.
3. Wrap your index and center fingers around both big toes, or place the palm of your hand on the interior or exterior of the foot.
4. Allow your hips to open as your knees melt down toward the earth; skull draw to lengthen the spine.
5. The ankles are directly above the knees but you can explore variations.

Modification

- Place a blanket under sacrum and/or neck.
- Use a strap around both feet.
- Practice one leg at a time.

SUPINE POSTURES

HALF HAPPY BABY (ARDHA ANANDA BALASANA)

Practicing Half Happy Baby will obtain a deeper release into the psoas and hip area. If back issues are present you will want to bend the foundational leg, keeping the sole of the foot on the earth. Hold for several breaths and switch legs.

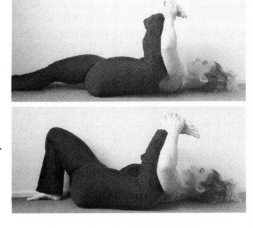

Deepen
- Straighten both legs without losing connection to the feet.
- Be sure the sacrum remains rooted into the earth.
- Rock from side to side.
- Attempt to connect the thigh to the earth for a deeper psoas stretch (Breathe).
- Use in a flow with Bridge or Wheel.

SUPINE LEG BEHIND HEAD (SUPTA BHAIRAVASANA)

Getting into the Posture

1. From a Seated Staff position, cradle or hug one leg into the torso to open the knee and hip.
2. Keep the opposite leg extended.
3. Tuck the shoulder (or tricep) under the cradled leg's knee; inch it up towards the shoulder as much as possible; place the ankle or foot on the back of the neck.
4. Bring both hands to heart center, on the ground, or on blocks.
5. Slowly lie back, keeping the foundational leg extended out long.

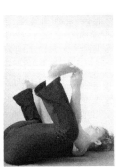

Modification
- Practice leg cradle.
- Keep leg on arm, don't bring upward to neck.
- Practice Half Happy Baby or Happy Baby.
- Practice Supine/Reclining Pigeon.
- Stay in Seated Leg Behind the Head.

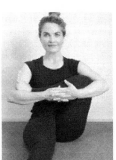 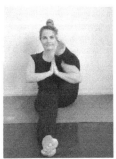 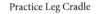

Practice Leg Cradle   Don't recline, foot anterior   Happy Baby

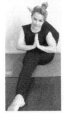 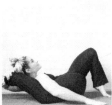 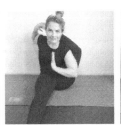 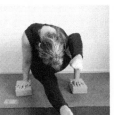 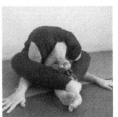

Inhale seated   Exhale recline   Leg behind head   Arm Balance   Turtle

Deepen
- Hold for several minutes before switching sides.
- Inhale to seated and exhale to recline.
- Hands to exterior of hips on ground for an arm balance.
- Place the foot behind the head.
- Practice Turtle.

Continue into a deeper expression by coming into...

YOGIC SLEEP POSE (YOGA NIDRASANA)

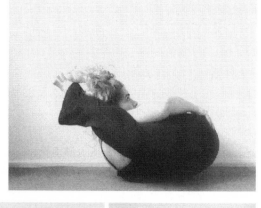

Getting into the Posture

1. Lying on your back, or from Supine Leg Behind Head, clasp each ankle with each hand bringing the knees down, slightly to the exterior of the torso.
2. Gently bring the knees into the armpits while your feet move toward the back of your head; allow your tailbone to be lifted off the earth here.
3. Place the hands on the outside of the heels as you lift your head off the ground.
4. Pull the shoulders through one at a time, so the knees move up and over the shoulders. A gentle rocking from side to side will help you achieve this.
5. Cross your ankles once they are behind your head to lock yourself in. Adjust your shoulders to be above the knees, and let your energy and breath settle in.
6. Final expression is to clasp the hands behind your low back.
7. Rest your head on your ankles.

Modification

- Place a blanket or hands under sacrum.
- Bend the knees.
- Practice Reclining Big Toe with or without a strap.
- Practice Half Happy Baby or Happy Baby.

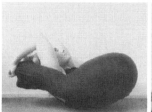 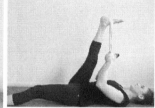

Arms above head　　　　Reclining Big Toe

When you lie down, you will not be afraid; when you lie down, your sleep will be sweet. Do not be afraid of sudden fear nor of the onslaught of the wicked when it comes, the Lord will be your confidence and will keep your foot from being caught. Proverbs 3:24-26

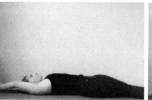 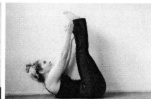

Half Happy Baby　　　　Happy Baby

DOUBLE LEG RAISES (URDHVA PRASARITA PADASANA)

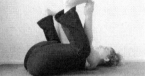

Getting into the Posture

1. From Legs up the Wall, extend arms long, biceps by ears with palms facing up; back of the hands are on the ground.
2. As you inhale, engage the lower abdominal.
3. As you exhale, with control, lower the legs as far as you can without compromising the abdominal and alignment. Movement can be slow or fast.

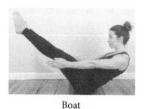

Modification

- Place a blanket or hands under sacrum.
- Bend the knees.
- Do classic crunches or practice Boat pose.

Boat

Deepen

- Slowly lower down 30 degrees, then 60 degrees, then hover a few inches off the earth.
- Can hold the hovering at the bottom, "scissor" the legs in and out, or "flutter" them up and down.
- Create a Vinyasa Flow with Plow.
- Both hands and feet connect in the center ("V-ups").

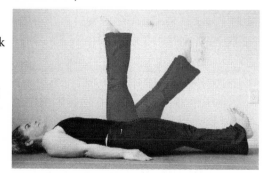

Practice "V-ups"

SUPINE POSTURES
RECLINING COUCH POSE (ANANTASANA)

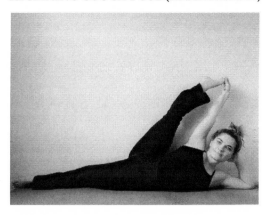

This is one of the only true side-facing poses. Technically, it's not a supine posture but it is really in a family by itself.

Getting into the Posture
1. Lying on one side, use your hand to prop up your head.
2. Bring the top leg up clasping the shin, ankle or toe.
3. Engage the core center as your breath is settled.

Modification
- Lessen the lateral flexion of the side stretch.
- Use a strap around the foot.

Deepen
- Each inhalation expands the rib cage slightly more and each exhalation will focus on deepening the posture.
- Flex the toes towards heart center, keeping the tops of thighs facing the sky energetically.
- You may also like pointing the toes, explore pointed and flexed to feel the differences.

Do not cast me away from Your presence and do not take Your Holy Spirit from me.
Restore to me the joy of Your salvation and sustain me with a willing spirit.
Then I will teach transgressors Your ways, and sinners will be converted to You. Psalm 51:11-13

Prayer:
Thank you Father, for guiding my mind, heart and the deepest parts of my soul into true and complete rest.
I surrender my will and ways; I throw in the towel and give up trying in my own "strength."
Here I am; speak to me now as I lay and bask in Your divine presence.

YOKED BREATH

So the Lord God formed the man from the dust of the ground, breathed life into his lungs, and the man became a living being. Genesis 2:7, International Standard Version

Our very breath is a gift from God. He formed us in His image, and His Spirit breathed life into us. Throughout your yoga practice, you can simply meditate on this truth. With every inhalation, bring in His presence, His Holy Spirit, and literally create space for Him. With every exhalation, think about getting rid of not only toxins from the physical body, but the emotional and spiritual body as well. Inhale Him; exhale you.

It's like anything else in life; we must get rid of old things to allow space for new things. If I don't clean and declutter the garage, then I can never park my car in it, let alone the new car I am dreaming about. Where will it go if I don't make space for it? If we are cluttered on the inside, where is space for God and His Spirit to work in and through us? You must find time to declutter and create room for Him. Create an environment for seeds He may want to plant, then give them space to grow and be birthed into existence.

This is what the Sovereign Lord says to these bones: I will make breath enter you, and you will come to life. Ezekiel 37:5

Then he said to me, "Prophesy to the breath; prophesy, son of man, and say to it, 'This is what the Sovereign Lord says: Come, breath, from the four winds and breathe into these slain, that they may live.'" So I prophesied as He commanded me, and breath entered them; they came to life and stood up on their feet—a vast army. Ezekiel 37:9-10

LET EVERYTHING THAT HAS BREATH PRAISE THE LORD! PRAISE THE LORD! Psalm 150:6

From scripture, we know that our very breath comes from God. He gives us life. His presence is your breath. Without Him, His presence, His Spirit, you have no life. No air. No breath. No purpose. YogaFaith allows you to come onto your mat, be still and know that He is God. Both literally and figuratively, He has given you *life!* Begin to focus on that precious gift of life: breath. In one inhalation and exhalation a miracle takes place.

HIS PRESENCE IS YOUR BREATH

Inspiration from the Holy Spirit can come in the form of inhalation. Biologically your respiratory system is working to oxygenate your blood. Spiritually your body is bringing in His presence. *Let every inhalation be your inspiration.* Invite the Holy Spirit in to cleanse every part of your life. All you ever have to do is invite Him *in.* I believe the Holy Spirit is the most ignored entity of the Trinity. He is all-powerful; do not forfeit this power that's available to you every day. After all, the Holy Spirit hovered over you and breathed air into you.

...He will give you another Comforter, and He will never leave you. He is the Holy Spirit, the Spirit who leads into all truth. The world at large cannot receive Him, for it isn't looking for Him and doesn't recognize Him. But you do, for He lives with you now and some day shall be in you. No, I will not abandon you or leave you as orphans in the storm—I will come to you. In just a little while I will be gone from the world, but I will still be present with you. John 14:15-19, The Living Bible

Inhalation creates space, physically, mentally, emotionally, and spiritually. Exhalation cleanses our body and spirit. Whether it's physically removing toxins, or another cleansing method, we rid ourselves of things that no longer belong in our lives. Breath is so very important as you practice YogaFaith and explore postures with your breath. Every inhalation will create space and every exhalation will allow you to go deeper into a posture.

Inhale those things that serve you and your destiny. Exhale those things that do not align with the Lord and your purpose.

THE HOLY SPIRIT HOVERED OVER YOU AND BREATHED AIR INTO YOU

DIG INTO THE WORD. YOUR SOUL WORK; GENESIS 2
A MEDITATION ON BREATH

God formed man out of dirt from the ground and blew into his nostrils the breath of life. The man came alive-a living soul! Genesis 2:7 The Message

Prayer:
Thank you Lord for the gift of breath! The very fact that my heart still beats and that I still breathe means you have something grand planned for me while I am alive on Earth! Thank you Holy Spirit for hovering over me and breathing inspiration into every cell and fiber of my being. With every breath that I take, I pray that it honors and glorifies You! In Jesus' mighty name, Amen!

GOD IS ENERGY

To this end I strenuously contend with all the energy Christ so powerfully works in me. Colossians 1:29

Knowing that Christ dwells within us, and His Holy Spirit guides us, we conclude that He gives us life, vitality, and energy. Colossians 1:29 says we contend with *all the energy that He so powerfully works in me.* Not *some* energy, not *weakly* works in us, but *powerfully* and *all* energy. This is great news. We cannot breathe without Him, and we will not be powerful or strengthened without Him.

And Moses said, "This is how you will know that the Lord has sent me to do all these things that I have done, for I have not done them on my own." Numbers 16:28

We cannot do anything in our own strength. We have to rely on God for everything, breath, life and, yes, our energy. He alone is our Source. God is the Creator of life; He is pure energy. Energy has a vibration, or a frequency. The further an organism is from its source, the lower its frequency and vibrations become. If we become cut off from this source, we die. The closer we are to the Source, God, the more alive we will be.

GOD IS LIGHT

We have heard from Him and announce to you, that God is Light, and in Him there is no darkness at all. If we say that we have fellowship with Him and yet walk in the darkness, we lie and do not practice the truth; but if we walk in the Light as He Himself is in the Light, we have fellowship with one another, and the blood of Jesus His Son cleanses us from all sin. If we say that we have no sin, we are deceiving ourselves and the truth is not in us. If we confess our sins, He is faithful and righteous to forgive us our sins and to cleanse us from all unrighteousness. If we say that we have not sinned, we make Him a liar and His word is not in us. 1 John 1:5-10

Even the darkness will not be dark to you; the night will shine like the day, for darkness is as light to you. Psalm 139:12

Come, descendants of Jacob, let us walk in the light of the Lord. Isaiah 2:5

He reveals deep and hidden things; He knows what lies in darkness, and light dwells with Him. Daniel 2:22

Again Jesus spoke to them, saying, "I am the light of the world. Whoever follows me will not walk in darkness, but will have the light of life." John 8:12

Do you follow Jesus? He promises you will have the light of life. Absorb that into your bones. If Christ dwells in us, then we are light also.

You are the light of the world. A town built on a hill cannot be hidden. Matthew 5:14

I encourage you to memorize a few of these scriptures. Doing so will help you spread His light through this ministry, Yoga-Faith, or your own personal ministry. Additionally, you'll realize that no matter what you go through, His promise is that it will never be in darkness. As you draw near to the True Source, you will increase your frequency and vibration and become *truly* alive!

ENERGY BODIES

Guard your heart with all vigilance, for from it are the sources of life. Proverbs 4:23

Think of your "energy body" as the electricity of your physical body. Without your energy body, your physical self could not function or survive. These energy bodies are the ethereal body (physical), the emotional body (heart), the mental body (mind), and the spiritual body (soul). When we received Christ, our spirits were made perfect. This is how God sees you, perfect and blameless. No matter the condition of your mind or physical body, your spirit is always perfect.

Our physical bodies contain a complex energy system that consists of energy centers and channels. Yoga philosophy describes our God-given energy centers as chakras. The energy channels, or nerves, that transport this vital energy throughout the body are known as nadis. The chakra system is a visual template used in the yoga world for understanding how to maintain spiritual, physical, emotional and social balance within one's body and others around us. Chakras correspond to vital points in the physical body, such as major networks of arteries, veins and nerves, similar to reflexology and acupuncture points.

The chakra system is a way for the yoga world to define what we as Christians know and believe to be true; God is our life force! The Holy Spirit breathes energy and life force into us. It is all because of Him that we have life!

The Sanskrit definition of chakra is "wheel," or "turning." This "wheel" is thought to spin and release vital energy, or life force, throughout the body. The Merriam-Webster Dictionary defines chakras as, "Any of several points of physical or spiritual energy in the human body." As believers in Christ, we know our physical bodies come from Him and the Holy Spirit breathes life and Spirit into our physical, as well as our spiritual bodies. The Father, Son and the Holy Spirit release vitality and all the life force necessary to live an abundant, fulfilled life through Christ. To Christians, this is known as the Trinity.

Paul writes:
Haven't you yet learned that your body is the home of the Holy Spirit God gave you, and that He lives within you? Your own body does not belong to you. For God has bought you with a great price. So use every part of your body to give glory back to God because He owns it.
1 Corinthians 6:19-20 The Living Bible

A BIBLICAL PICTURE OF MAN
A THREE-PART WHOLE (1 THESSALONIANS 5:23)

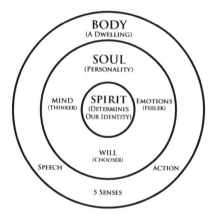

The Holy Spirit dwells within those who have received salvation. This life force within us is from God Himself, it is His Spirit. Because our physical body is God's holy temple, our postures of prayer will glorify Christ who created us and gave us life itself. As we use our physical body to worship the Lord, our spirit connects with God's Spirit in a powerful yet intimate space. The energy and sacredness of this Divine dialogue is unlike any other worship.

David wrote:
You, God, are my God, earnestly I seek You; I thirst for You, my whole being longs for You. Psalm 63:1

He writes of his whole being longing for God. I personally do not know how else to interpret this and so many other scriptures like it, other than to worship the Lord with all of me. My physical body, my spiritual body, my mind and my soul. This is whole worship, with all of my energy.

OUR GOD-GIVEN ENERGY CENTERS

Let's dive deeper into how parallel the Chakra system is to the Word of God.

There are seven God-given energy centers throughout our system known as Chakras. We will start at the top of the head and work our way down to the base of the spine.

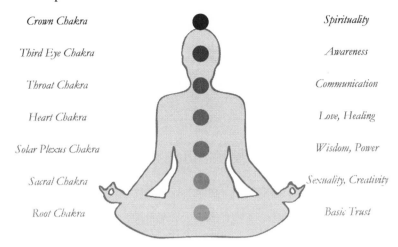

Crown Chakra	*Spirituality*
Third Eye Chakra	*Awareness*
Throat Chakra	*Communication*
Heart Chakra	*Love, Healing*
Solar Plexus Chakra	*Wisdom, Power*
Sacral Chakra	*Sexuality, Creativity*
Root Chakra	*Basic Trust*

CHAKRA 7: CROWN CHAKRA, THOUGHT. "I UNDERSTAND."
THE CONNECTION TO YOUR DIVINE PURPOSE AND SPIRITUALITY

Get wisdom, get understanding...Do not forsake wisdom, and she will protect you.
The beginning of wisdom is this: Get wisdom. Though it cost all you have, get understanding. Proverbs 4:5-7

This is known as the crown chakra that relates to consciousness as pure awareness. It is our connection to the greater world beyond our earthly world and the one we see with our fleshly eyes. Being one with Christ and His spirit allows our spiritual eyes to see. Those who are not of the Spirit, do not have "spiritual eyes", they cannot see spiritual things, it is impossible. Through the Holy Spirit's guidance, this energy center that Christ created, brings us knowledge, wisdom, understanding, spiritual connection and the realization that we have all power working within us, it began the day we received Christ as our personal Savior.

I will give you hidden treasures, riches stored in secret places, so that you may know that I am the Lord,
the God of Israel, who summons you by name. Isaiah 45:3

God tells us that His thoughts are not our thoughts, and our thoughts are not His. (Hallelujah and Amen!) As we become yoked to Christ, He promises to reveal hidden mysteries, wonders and treasures. There are many great and mighty secrets that we can know just by drawing close to Christ. As we get to the secret place of the most High, our spiritual eyes become fully awakened and there are actually no secrets there in the secret place, we just have to get there. As we praise Him, He blasts us with wisdom and knowledge. As soon as we praise Him, Isaiah 45:3 will begin to manifest. Remember when Jehoshaphat praised Him in 2 Chronicles 20? Scripture tells us *as soon* as the praise left their mouth, God *immediately* set ambushes against their enemies. So much begins to happen in the spiritual and earthly realms as we begin to praise. Our all-knowing infinite God downloads wisdom and knowledge into our thoughts, intellect and emotions, what the yoga world describes as the thought chakra. Meditate on the Creator of your amazing brain, wisdom and knowledge.

CHAKRA 6: THIRD EYE CHAKRA. LIGHT. "I SEE."
BRAIN, EYES, EARS, NOSE, PINEAL GLAND
AND CENTER OF INTUITION

I pray that the eyes of your heart may be enlightened in order that you may know the hope to which He has called you,
the riches of His glorious inheritance in His holy people. Ephesians 1:18

This chakra is known as the brow chakra or third eye center. It is related to the act of seeing, both physically and intuitively. It awakens our understanding and allows us to see clearly and have a healthy perspective on life. With a Christ centered practice, we see the blessing in everything and everybody. We freely receive grace and begin to freely extend grace to others. As we draw closer to the heart of God, we begin to have an eternal perspective. The things that used to seem like big problems, become smaller as we magnify God. To magnify means to enlarge. As we enlarge Christ, everything else becomes smaller and burns off of our lives.

I have seen the task which God has given the sons of men with which to occupy themselves. He has made everything appropriate in its time. He has also set eternity in their heart, yet so that man will not find out the work which God has done from the beginning even to the end. I know that there is nothing better for them than to rejoice and to do good in one's lifetime. Ecclesiastes 3:10-12

We may not always know the answer or be able to see the full scope of what lies ahead, we only need to know the One that knows all the answers and sees it all!

Chakra 5: Throat Chakra, SOUND, "I speak."
THYROID, TRACHEA, THROAT, MOUTH; INNER MAN AND CREATIVE IDENTITY

Speak to us and we will listen.
But do not have God speak to us or we will die. Exodus 20:19

Come to me with your ears wide open. Listen, and you will find life. I will make an everlasting covenant with you. I will give you all the unfailing love I promised to David. Isaiah 55:3

This is the God given energy center located in the throat and related to communication and creativity. The great thing about YogaFaith is that you create intimate time with Christ, and begin to make it a priority. How can we hear from God if we do not take time to open our ears and listen. How will we know what to speak and share with others, if we are not asking Him to put words in our mouth, show us the way or speak into our hearts and minds?

Do you have eyes but fail to see, and ears but fail to hear? Mark 8:18

Some will never be able to perceive what the Lord is saying and doing, they physically and spiritually cannot hear.

They have mouths, but they do not speak. They have eyes, but they do not see. They have ears, but they do not hear, nor is there any breath at all in their mouths. Psalm 135:16-17

God has blessed each and every one with specific talents and gifts that we must use to glorify Him while living out the plans and purposes that He has for us. We must have the ears to hear what He is calling His children to do on the earth today.
You may have heard the saying that the two most important days are the day you were born and the day you find out why you were born. There is nothing more frustrating than doing something you were never meant to do. We all have seasons where we cry out to God, "Why was I born? What do you want me to do? What on Earth am I supposed to be doing?" The sooner you find out why you were born, the longer you can use your talents for eternal purposes.

He has filled him with the Spirit of God, in wisdom, understanding, knowledge and in all craftsmanship; to make designs...so as to perform in every inventive work. He also has put in his heart to teach...He has filled them with skill to perform every work of an engraver, a designer and embroiderer, as performers of every work and maker of every design. Exodus 35:34-35

Chakra 4: Heart Chakra, AIR. "I love."
HEART, LUNGS, SHOULDERS, RIBS, BREAST, DIAPHRAGM; IDENTITY IN CHRIST AND SELF-ACCEPTANCE

And the peace of God, which transcends all understanding, will guard your hearts and minds. Philippians 4:7

I think this may be the most powerful energy center that God created in our body. Known as the heart chakra, it is related to love, and God is love. He has created us to love deeply, feel compassion and empathy and be as gracious and loving to others as He has been toward us. When our heart is healthy and we realize our true identity in Christ, we have a peace that passes all understanding and a joy that this world cannot give nor take away!

Strive for full restoration, encourage one another, be of one mind, live in peace. And the God of love and peace will be with you. 2 Corinthians 13:11

Our thoughts, emotions and actions are all powered by love, so we want to continually check in with our heart and make sure we are keeping it clear of all junk. Any walls that have been built, any bitterness, an offense, any unforgiveness, we must daily renew and cleanse ourselves from all of these things.

And He has given us this command:
> *Anyone who loves God must also love their brother and sister.* 1 John 4:21

Whoever confesses that Jesus is the Son of God, God abides in him, and he in God. We have come to know and have believed the love which God has for us. God is love, and the one who abides in love abides in God, and God abides in him. By this, love is perfected with us, so that we may have confidence in the day of judgment; because as He is, so also are we in this world. 1 John 4:15-17

He predestined us to adoption as sons through Jesus Christ to Himself, according to the kind intention of His will, oh the praise of the glory of His grace, which He freely bestowed on us in the Beloved. In Him we have redemption through His blood, the forgiveness of our trespasses, according to the riches of His grace. Ephesians 1:5-7

Isn't love powerful? The next time you get stingy with your grace and love, remember what God went through to save, redeem, forgive and love you.

CHAKRA 3: SOLAR PLEXUS CHAKRA, FIRE, "I DO."
ABDOMEN, LIVER, GALLBLADDER, STOMACH, KIDNEYS;
POWER AND EGO (EXHALE EGO)

Putting aside all filthiness and all that remains of wickedness, in humility receive the word implanted, which is able to save your souls. But prove yourselves doers of the word, and not merely hearers who delude themselves. For if anyone is a hearer of the word and not a doer, he is like a man who looks at his natural face in a mirror; for once he has looked at himself and gone away, he has immediately forgotten what kind of person he was. James 1:21-24

It is Christ working in us that makes us strong. He says that in our weakness His strength is perfected. This life force epicenter is known as the power chakra. It is located in the solar plexus and is associated with governing our personal power, will, autonomy, as well as our digestion and metabolism. Because of it's location, deep folds and revolved postures will cleanse and detox your internal organs and keep everything flowing and healthy.

Today I have given you the choice between life and death, between blessings and curses. Now I call on heaven and earth to witness the choice you make. Oh, that you would choose life, so that you and your descendants might live!
Deuteronomy 30:19 New Living Translation

God always gives us the power to choose.

We can let go of our ego and rely on God for absolutely everything. The world may say ego, but God says humility. The world may seek to self serve, but we are to be Christ-like and serve others. If you always feel like a fish swimming upstream, that is because God is doing work in you. It's uncomfortable at first, but as His power, grace, strength and love consume you, His ways become second nature.

You experience the love of Christ, though it is too great to understand fully. Then you will be made complete with all the fullness of life and power that comes from God. Ephesians 3:19

CHAKRA 2: SACRAL CHAKRA, WATER. "I FEEL."
ABDOMEN, GENITALS, WOMB, PELVIS, APPENDIX;
EMOTIONS AND RELATIONSHIPS

I give you a new command: Love one another. Just as I have loved you, you must also love one another. John 13:34

Located in the abdomen, lower back and sexual organs, this powerful God-given life center relates to emotions, relations and sexuality. It connects us to others through feeling, desire, sensation and movement. It brings us fluidity, grace, depth of feeling, fulfillment and the ability to accept change. This life center is also associated with water because of the elements of fluidity and grace.

One thing is constant and that is change. That is why it so important to remain pliable. The vision and our True North never changes, but sometimes the route, package or vehicle may change. It is also important to journey with like-minded people that are striving towards a common goal and destination. I ask you, who is on your plane? Are you traveling with the right people? Are they supposed to be going with you, is everyone going to the same destination? These are very important questions. Our inner circle and who we do life with is extremely important. God will send people for your life to help you fulfill your purpose, it maybe for a short, long or permanent season.

We want to treat all people as Christ demands us to in John 13:34. We are fairly good at treating people good that are similar to us or kind to us. It's when others are different, look different, believe different and even smell different that we sometimes forget the love and grace that was freely poured upon us.

But He said to me, "My grace is sufficient for you, for my power is made perfect in weakness." Therefore I will boast all the more gladly about my weaknesses, so that Christ's power may rest on me. 2 Corinthians 12:9

CHAKRA 1: BASE OR ROOT CENTER. EARTH, "I AM." PHYSICAL BODY SUPPORT, BLOOD, IMMUNE SYSTEM; SECURITY, FAMILY AND TRUE IDENTITY

Put your trust in the Lord your God and you will be established. Put your trust in His prophets and succeed. 2 Chronicles 20:20

If it is so that you continue in the faith, grounded and steadfast, and not moved away from the hope of the Good News which you heard, which is being proclaimed in all creation under heaven; of which I, Paul, was made a servant. Colossians 1:23

Located at the base of the spine, this is the God given core power that forms the foundation of our energy, strength and ability to act. It represents the elements that are associated to earth and relates to our survival instincts, sense of grounding, connection to our bodies as well as the physical plane. It is the center of our emotional and physical health. When healthy with God's life force flowing through us, we are able to make wise and sound decisions, obtain overall health, prosperity, (wholeness; nothing missing, broken or lacking) security, as well as the powerful presence of God overflowing and extending outwardly.

That Christ may dwell in your hearts through faith, that you, being rooted and grounded in love. Ephesians 3:17

We are to be doers of the word and act upon what we know. Our obedience is an act of sacrifice and worship. We are able to do anything, for it is God that has graced us to do all things pertaining to life.

I can do all things through Him who strengthens me. Philippians 4:13

We know that any success is through Him and not in our own strength, otherwise we would all be up a creek! Through Him. He says, "I am the great I am." We can never be the, "I am." Oh, isn't it grand that we just need to *know* the Great I Am?

God replied to Moses, "I Am Who I Am. Say this to the people of Israel: I Am has sent me to you." Exodus 3:14

GOD CREATED ENERGY

Did you know that when we get to Heaven His glory is our light source? No longer will you need the sun to shine by day, nor the moon to give its light by night, for the Lord your God will be your everlasting light and your God will be your glory (Isaiah 60:19).

And the city has no need of sun or moon, for the glory of God illuminates the city, and the Lamb is its light. Revelation 21:23

God is energy. He is everything. He is Spirit. He is love. He is mercy. He is our Father. He is omniscient, and so much more. There is no denying that we are energy beings, we are also spiritual beings. I am not saying that we are 'just' energy, or that God is 'just' energy. Energy is just one part that makes us fearfully and wonderfully created.

Each one of our energy centers, or pressure points, relates to certain life issues, organs and specific glands. Many times we trap tension and trauma in various locations. When you learn of these locations, you can practice strategies that can heal from an internal place, and with the Lord, you will find true and lasting healing. Restorative yoga postures, pressure points, energy centers and essential oils combined with the power of Christ can heal any disease, ailment or trauma. See the following reflexology charts for one example of how the knowledge of certain locations can help you in your healing journey.

Praise the Lord, oh my soul;
all my inmost being,
praise His holy name.

Praise the Lord, oh my soul,
and forget not all his benefits,

Who forgives all your sins
and heals all your diseases,

Who redeems your life from the pit
and crowns you with
love and compassion,

Who satisfies your desires with good
things so that your youth is
renewed like the eagle's.

Psalm 103:1-5

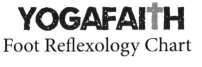
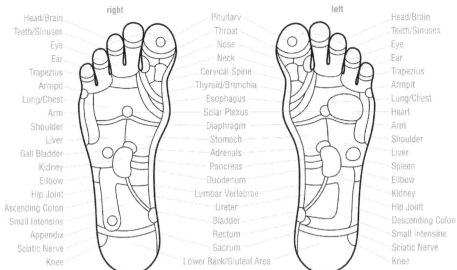

Foot Reflexology Chart

right
Head/Brain, Teeth/Sinuses, Eye, Ear, Trapezius, Armpit, Lung/Chest, Arm, Shoulder, Liver, Gall Bladder, Kidney, Elbow, Hip Joint, Ascending Colon, Small Intensine, Appendix, Sciatic Nerve, Knee

center: Pituitary, Throat, Nose, Neck, Cervical Spine, Thyroid/Bronchia, Esophagus, Solar Plexus, Diaphragm, Stomach, Adrenals, Pancreas, Duodenum, Lumbar Vertebrae, Ureter, Bladder, Rectum, Sacrum, Lower Back/Gluteal Area

left
Head/Brain, Teeth/Sinuses, Eye, Ear, Trapezius, Armpit, Lung/Chest, Heart, Arm, Shoulder, Liver, Spleen, Elbow, Kidney, Hip Joint, Descending Colon, Small Intensine, Sciatic Nerve, Knee

You are the One who created my
innermost parts; You knit me together
while I was still in my mother's womb.

I give thanks to You that I was
marvelously set apart. Your works are
wonderful, I know that very well.

My bones weren't hidden from You when
I was being put together in a secret place,
when I was being woven together in the
deep parts of the earth.

Your eyes saw my embryo, and on Your
scroll every day was written that was
being formed for me, before any one of
them had yet happened.

God, Your plans are incomprehensible to
me! Their total number is countless!

Psalm 139:13-17 (Common English Bible)

Hand Reflexology Chart

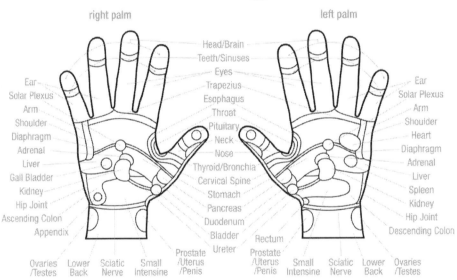

right palm
Ear, Solar Plexus, Arm, Shoulder, Diaphragm, Adrenal, Liver, Gall Bladder, Kidney, Hip Joint, Ascending Colon, Appendix

center: Head/Brain, Teeth/Sinuses, Eyes, Trapezius, Esophagus, Throat, Pituitary, Neck, Nose, Thyroid/Bronchia, Cervical Spine, Stomach, Pancreas, Duodenum, Bladder, Ureter, Rectum

bottom: Ovaries/Testes, Lower Back, Sciatic Nerve, Small Intensine, Prostate/Uterus/Penis, Prostate/Uterus/Penis, Small Intensine, Sciatic Nerve, Lower Back, Ovaries/Testes

left palm
Ear, Solar Plexus, Arm, Shoulder, Heart, Diaphragm, Adrenal, Liver, Spleen, Kidney, Hip Joint, Descending Colon

Source: YogaFaith.org

Emotional or physical tensions and/or trauma, such as abuse we may not even remember, could be trapped deep in our core. This can block energy and life. For example, have you ever held an offense, harbored bitterness, or been unable to forgive? When you surrender that, you will experience an enormous release, and life will "flow" again. This is what it feels like to unblock part of our life or a specific area in our body. We want to give all this junk and garbage to God. Surrender it completely, finally, so your life can flow freely. Just as God is light, we as His children should also be light. You are the light of the world. A city set on a hill that cannot be hidden, nor does anyone light a lamp and put it under a basket, but on the lamp stand, and it gives light to all who are in the house (Matt. 5:14-15).

Let your light shine before men in such a way that they may see your good works, and glorify your Father who is in heaven.
Matthew 5:16

Freely you have received; freely give. Matthew 10:8

Prayer:
Thank you Father for creating life! I praise You that I am fearfully and intricately made in the image of Your Son. I thank You for Your Holy Spirit guiding me into all truth and dwelling within me so that I thrive with the abundant life You promised. Amen!

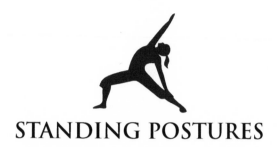

STANDING POSTURES

Remain alert. Keep standing firm in your faith. Keep on being courageous and strong.
1 Corinthians 16:13 International Standard Version

So that Christ may dwell in your hearts through faith; and that you, being rooted and grounded in love, may be able to comprehend with all the saints what is the breadth and length and height and depth, and to know the love of Christ which surpasses knowledge, that you may be filled up to all the fullness of God. Ephesians 3:17-18 King James Version

Scripture reveals that God's strength is perfected in our weakness. "But He said to me, 'My grace is sufficient for you, for my power is made perfect in weakness.' Therefore I will boast all the more gladly about my weaknesses, so that Christ's power may rest on me." (2 Corinthians 12:9). Would you take a moment and let that settle into your bones and spirit?

If we operate in our own strength, in reality, it is not strength at all. We operate in complete weakness without the Lord's help. Our flesh is weak; it always has been and always will be. Relying on God's strength is a throughout-the-day kind of renewal. We are always weak. I want you to understand that in your weakness, which is every day, His strength is perfected. This is a powerful truth. Knowing this, we can always stand firm in His strength, which means we are never weak. Is this mind-blowing or what?

When did you last feel weak, weary, or flat-out exhausted? Chances are, it wasn't that long ago; maybe it is right now. The good news is that your Father, the Creator of the Universe and galaxies (you know, the One who created you and knows you intimately), is all-powerful and never runs out of strength. He never runs out of strength! Today, I encourage you to draw on His strength. Exhale your weaknesses, and inhale His might.

I simply love The Message's version of what Paul writes in 2 Corinthians 12:7-10:

I was given the gift of a handicap to keep me in constant touch with my limitations. Satan's angel did his best to get me down; what he in fact did was push me to my knees. No danger then of walking around high and mighty! At first I didn't think of it as a gift, and begged God to remove it. Three times I did that, and then He told me, My grace is enough; it's all you need. "My strength comes into its own in your weakness." Once I heard that, I was glad to let it happen. I quit focusing on the handicap and began appreciating the gift. It was a case of Christ's strength moving in on my weakness. Now I take limitations in stride, and with good cheer, these limitations that cut me down to size—abuse, accidents, opposition, bad breaks, I just let Christ take over! And so the weaker I get, the stronger I become.

Did you catch this? "The weaker I get, the stronger I become." Wow! Paul is saying that God's grace and His strength is all we ever need. You do not need to worry about anything, including your weaknesses or handicaps.

Isaiah predates Paul's passage in Isaiah 40:31, which The Message translates eloquently. Meditate on this beautiful passage as it correlates to your strength as well as strong, standing yoga postures.

Why would you ever complain, O Jacob, (replace your name here) or, whine, Israel, saying, "God has lost track of me. He doesn't care what happens to me"? Don't you know anything? Haven't you been listening? God doesn't come and go. God lasts. He's Creator of all you can see or imagine. He doesn't get tired out, doesn't pause to catch His breath. And He knows everything, inside and out. He energizes those who get tired, gives fresh strength to dropouts. For even young people tire and drop out, young folk in their prime stumble and fall. But those who wait upon God get fresh strength. They spread their wings and soar like eagles, they run and don't get tired, they walk and don't lag behind.

Do not let the enemy of this world steal your energy or strength for one more second! Your Father is waiting for you to call upon Him, need Him and prove His power in your life! Perhaps you are fatigued. Simply write these few lines down and place them where you'll see them as an everyday reminder that you, operating in Him, are strong.

He doesn't get tired out, doesn't pause to catch His breath, He energizes those who get tired, gives fresh strength... Isaiah 40:31 The Message

In yoga, you may hear "root down to rise up." It comes from various philosophies, but we can anchor it in God's Word and the truth of Ephesians 3:17-18 (above), being rooted and grounded in Him. In any standing or balancing postures, when you connect all four corners of both feet to the earth, that is "being rooted." Then, when you extend your arms, also known as your "branches," this is where yogis derive, "root down to rise up." Isn't it amazing to be rooted in Christ so you are strong in His might?

Are you ready to improve your strength through Him? You will enjoy the benefits of standing postures. They remind us that outside of Him and His will, we are weak. While practicing your standing postures, meditate on His never-ending strength and power. Call upon Him whenever you need to. He is always there; He's ready to make you your strongest even when you are at your weakest.

Standing postures are the foundation of all other yoga poses. Standing poses help us to not only develop greater physical strength, stamina, flexibility, endurance, and balance, but also improve mental clarity, focus, concentration, determination, willpower and memory.

Standing poses are good for your posture in general, as they improve and strengthen the stabilizing muscles. While improving our posture, we learn how to correct structural problems. These postures teach our spine to align, extend, move, properly function and rotate safely in all directions. Standing postures facilitate effective circulation, digestion, mobility and overall physical awareness. Because standing poses improve balance, your feet, legs, joints and muscles will be strengthened. In addition to strengthening your legs and other muscles, each posture will stretch and lengthen different areas of the body and increase flexibility, stamina and endurance.

You can incorporate back bends and revolved postures into standing postures, to stretch and strengthen muscles and joints throughout the entire body. Any back bend or side bend relies on strength and complete engagement of the lower body. Standing postures develop strength and stamina to assist with back-bending poses. These postures will develop concentration and muscle strength to master other challenging postures. You will move through all directional planes and axes with standing postures. You will develop keen body awareness and God-confidence in your body image as you become whole; mind, body and spirit.

While the following postures are the foundation of all other postures, you may need patience as you master them. Remember to embrace the journey. Like our walk with the Lord, it is all a journey, a faith walk if you will. Never grow weary of being persistent. Also, each side of your body is different from the other. You may find that one side is easier than the other; this is normal. A past injury may creep into your practice that throws your balance off. That is when standing postures may help you, not just in your yoga practice, but also to use the endurance, concentration, and other skills you develop in these poses in your everyday life. Yoga is much more than stretching. It is a wholeness practice. Center your practice on Christ, and you have everything you need to live in an abundance of wholeness and strength.

Benefits of standing postures include, but are not limited to:
- Strengthens and tones the abdomen, lower body, especially the legs and buttocks.
- Strengthens the back muscles, improves alignment of the spine improving posture.
- Strengthens shoulders, chest and arms.
- Stretches and opens hips, groin and chest.
- Therapeutic for mild sciatica, flat feet, backache, indigestion and asthma.
- Standing hip openers and wide squats can be therapeutic for pregnancy, opening the pelvic region and preparing the body for childbirth.
- Improves concentration, mental focus and relieves mild depression.
- Revitalizing, strengthening and stimulating.

Cautions include, but are not limited to:
- Severe back issues such as a herniated disk.
- High or low blood pressure, shoulder, back and neck injury - practice modifications.
- Foot or knee injury.
- Headache or migraine, vertigo, glaucoma or sinusitis.
- Avoid deep bends and twists if pregnancy, diarrhea, ulcer or severe asthma exists.

Stand firm. Let nothing move you. Always give yourselves fully to the work of the Lord, because you know that your labor in the Lord is not in vain. 1 Corinthians 15:58

DIG INTO THE WORD. YOUR SOUL WORK; 1 CORINTHIANS 15
THE MESSAGE BIBLE
A MEDITATION ON STANDING POSTURES

THE POSTURES

MOUNTAIN POSE (TADASANA)

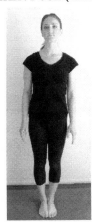

Preparatory Pose
- Child's Pose or Resting Angel
- Standing Forward Fold
- Downward Facing Dog, High or Low Plank

Getting into the Posture
1. Feet can be together or hip-width apart.
2. All four corners of both feet are rooted into the earth.
3. Engage both legs; rotate femurs inward.
4. Slightly tuck your sacrum under.
5. Shoulders are away from ears.
6. Gaze is forward; spine is long.

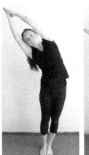 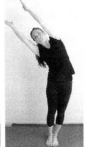 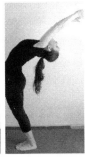 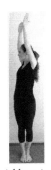

Use a wall, chair, and/or props

Modification
- Keep hands by side.
- Sit on edge of chair, and lengthen spine. Practice with blocks under feet.
- Use a wall; heels and sacrum should touch but not head.

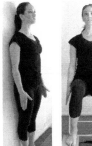 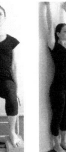 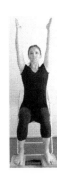

Add lateral flexion   Add a back bend   Add a twist
(Standing Half Crescent)

Deepen
- Raise arms above head; interlace fingers, and press palms up.
- Close your eyes.
- Incorporate a back bend or twist from the torso side to side.
- Raise arms; tilt side to side (lateral flexion). This is Standing Half Crescent/Crescent Moon (Chandrasana); legs can be together or hip-width apart.
- Practice arm variations.

UPWARD SALUTE (URDHVA HASTASANA)

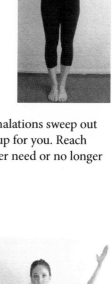

Getting into the Posture

1. From Mountain Pose, extend arms upward. Create space between the shoulders and ears by pulling the scapulas back and downward.
2. With the arms raised, biceps near the ears, energetically pull the arms backward as you root down in the feet and engage the legs.

Modification

- Keep hands by side (Mountain).
- Sit on edge of chair, lengthen spine, and raise hands.
- Stand against a wall.

Deepen

- See Deepen for previous posture, Mountain Pose.

Counter Poses

Integrate all the grounded and balancing sensations from Mountain, Standing Crescent and Upward Salute throughout all your standing postures. Enjoy the security of being firmly grounded and stable in Christ. Exhalations sweep out insecurities and worries; inhalations bring in security and courage. Inhalations reach for everything that is stored up for you. Reach for the new season and the new beginnings, while exhalations expel the "old." Exhale away everything you no longer need or no longer serves you. Inhale, reaching for the new life.

I came to give you life, and that life more abundantly. John 10:10

GODDESS POSE (UTKATA KONASANA)

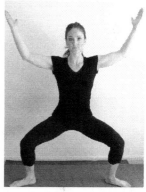

Getting into the Posture

1. Position your legs approximately three feet apart.
2. Feet face out about 45 degrees.
3. Raise elbows to shoulder height. Hands are upward, palms facing in. Arms remain active, as if you are holding a beach ball.
4. Bending both knees, the tailbone sinks down towards the earth.

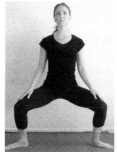 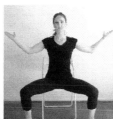

Modification

- Keep hands by side.
- Sit on edge of chair, focusing on lengthening the spine.

Keep arms low   Use a chair

Deepen

- Raise arms above head.
- Deepen squat.
- Close your eyes.
- Let your exhalations take your tailbone closer to the earth as you continue to lift through the heart and stay buoyant, resilient.

Inhale strength, courage and determination as you continue to exhale pride, ego and loftiness. Inhale Him; exhale you. He must increase as you decrease.

STANDING FORWARD FOLD (UTTANASANA)

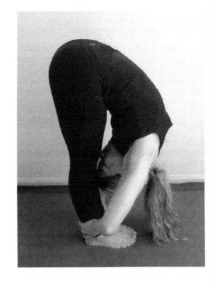

Getting into the Posture

1. From Mountain Pose, feet are together or hip-width apart. Raise arms if desired; lengthen the torso.
2. Hinging at the hips, fold torso down. Bend your knees as much as you need to.
3. Press your heels into the earth.
4. Continue to "sandwich" yourself in by bringing your torso closer to your thighs.

Modification

- Use blocks under both hands and elevate the spine.
- Use a strap under the arches of your feet, and hold the strap instead of your toes.
- Bend the knees as much as needed.
- Practice using a chair.
- Practice Standing Half Forward Fold (Ardha Uttanasana).

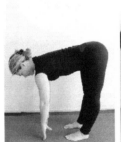
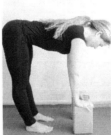
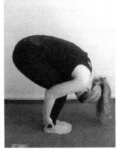
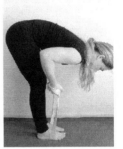

Half Forward Fold   Add blocks   Bend knees   Add strap

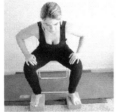
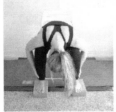
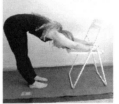

Lessen the fold   Practice with chair and blocks   Rest on chair seat

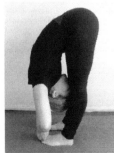
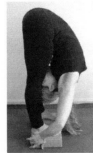

Forehead to knee   Stand on blocks

Deepen

- Continue to use your breath to work on a deeper hinging at the hips so your gaze continues to reach the forehead closer to shins.
- Tuck the chin into the chest, allowing elbows to bend deeper as the top of your head comes closer to ground.
- Stand on blocks and deepen fold.

To deepen further, practice…

HALF BOUND LOTUS FORWARD FOLD (ARDHA BADDHA PADMOTTANASANA)

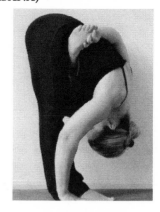

Place one foot into the crease of the opposite hip before forward folding to practice Half Lotus Forward Fold.

Exhalations allow you to "let it all go," releasing anything that holds you back from God's greatness. Let it all hang heavy; your exhalation continue to release any heavy burdens. Inhale, lengthen the spine and create space for the new air, breath and season.

Inhale, becoming lighter and lighter as you release things you were never intended to carry on your back. Allow the Lord to speak to you and "gather in" a new perspective in this posture.

Deepening even further, practice…

BIG TOE POSE (PADANGUSTHASANA)

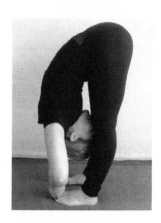

Getting into the Posture
1. From Standing Forward Fold, separate your feet about six inches or hip-width apart.
2. Wrap your index and middle finger ("peace fingers") around the big toes.
3. Lengthen through the torso, with your head and torso moving together.
4. On your inhalations, find length in the spine without impinging your neck by looking up.
5. Straighten out the arms, as you exhale, elbows come out towards the sides. Allow your head to hang heavy.
6. Hips are directly above the ankles; heels press into the earth. Breathe into the hamstrings.

Modification
- Use blocks or a chair under both hands to elevate the spine.
- Use a strap under arches of feet and hold strap instead of toes.
- Stay in Seated Forward Fold; you can use a blanket under knees and/or sacrum.

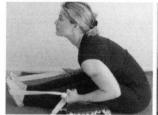
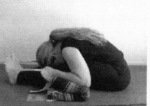
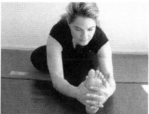

Strap and blanket under knees | Bend forward | Seated Forward Fold one foot at a time

Deepen
- Continue to use your breath to work on a deeper hinging at the hips reaching, perhaps connecting.
- Tuck chin in towards the chest and gaze at the navel, massaging the thyroid and parathyroid gland to increase metabolism.
- Press all four corners of feet into the earth as you lift both thighs towards the sky.
- Allow both elbows to bend deeper as the top of your head comes closer to ground and the forehead closer to the shins.

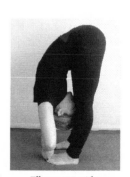

Elbows out wide, forehead to knees

Your exhalations let it all go as you "hang up" things you no longer have space for. Now that you have created space as you exhale, your inhalations bring in the things and people that God has for your life. Find what your body, mind and spirit crave in this posture. Feel secure, balanced and stable in your deepest expression of this posture. Settle in and breathe.

WIDE-LEGGED FORWARD FOLD (PRASARITA PADOTTANASANA)

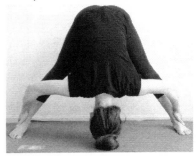

Getting into the Posture

1. From Mountain Pose, step one foot wide, approximately three feet or more.
2. "Airplane" your arms out to the sides and hinge forward from the hips.
3. Place your hands in the center, on a block(s), or reach to the exterior of the ankles.
(You may need to adjust your stance once you get into the forward fold. Widen your stance or try turning the toes inward for a deeper hamstring stretch.)
4. Allow the crown of your head to sink closer to the floor with every breath.
5. You may want to pull your forehead to the ground as opposed to the crown. See what works for you. If you practice forehead to ground, use caution not to injure your neck. Never force anything.

Modification

- Use blocks under both hands to elevate the spine.
- Use a strap under arches of feet and hold strap instead of toes/ankles.
- Place forearms on the seat of chair or bench.
- Rest crown of head on a block or bolster.

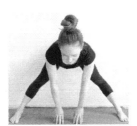
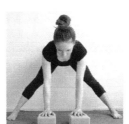
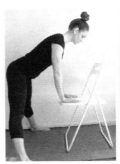

Lessen the hinge   Use blocks   Use chair   Rest on seat

Deepen

- Continue to use your breath to work on a deeper hinging at the hips so gaze continues to reach the forehead closer to shins and beyond legs, someday.
- Press all four corners of both feet into the earth as you lift both thighs towards the sky.
- Allow both elbows to bend deeper as the top of your head comes closer to ground.
- Rolling shoulder blades back and down, place hands in a backward prayer position, (Seal Salutation/ Rear Anjali Mudra), fingertips pointing toward your head pinky fingers touch and then come into a deeper forward fold.
- Practice Tripod Headstand.
- You may add a twist to this posture, coming into Revolved Wide-Legged Forward Fold.

To further deepen the posture practice…

REVOLVED WIDE-LEGGED FORWARD FOLD (PARIVRTTA PRASARITA PADOTTANASANA)

Getting into the Posture

1. From Wide Legged Forward Fold, grasp one hand to opposite ankle or directly in front and mid center to the body.
2. Open shoulder and chest upward as you outstretch opposite hand.

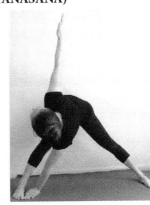

Inhale calm; exhale chaos. Inhale cleansing and renewal; exhale toxins and things that are no longer alive in your life. Allow yourself to surrender in your deepest expression of this posture, perhaps moving into a headstand or simply staying still. Be open to a new perspective on things that have caused worry or anxiety. Give it all to God here.

LOW LUNGE (ANJANEYASANA)

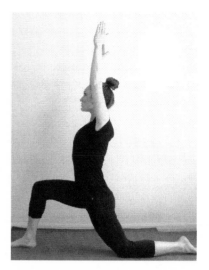

Getting into the Posture

1. From Mountain pose, gently place one knee on a cushion or your mat.
2. The opposite leg bends out in front of you.
3. Hands can be placed at hips, on the ground, on blocks or extended, wherever you find a comfortable place that you can focus on the hips opening.

Modification

- Roll a blanket or a similar prop to place under back knee.
- Use the seat of a chair to rest forearms on or simply hold chair.
- Place hands at hips, heart center or tallest height of blocks.

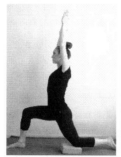 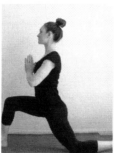 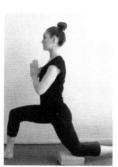

Rest back knee on   Keep arms down   Practice both
a block

Deepen

- Raise arms above head, drawing the shoulder blades down.
- Include a back bend with arms lifted.
- Interlace fingers behind back, opening up the chest and look up.
- Continue to focus on opening up the hip and groin area with each breath.
- Add back bends or side bends to this pose.

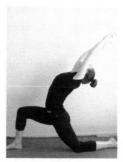

Add a back bend

Allow every inhalation to increase openness and vulnerability. Every exhalation sends out mistrust and pride. Inhale surrender, exhale ego. Inhale peace, exhale conflict.

Peace I leave with you; my peace I give to you. Not as the world gives do I give to you.
Let not your hearts be troubled, neither let them be afraid. John 14:27

To further deepen the posture, lift the back knee off the ground to practice...

HIGH LUNGE / CRESCENT (ALANASANA)

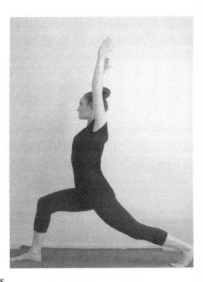

Getting into the Posture
1. From Mountain Pose, step one foot back, both feet face forward.
2. The front leg lunges, someday the front thigh parallel to the earth (Be sure to not let the knee extend past the ankle).
3. The back leg is energetically lifting towards the sky.
4. The toes of the back foot are on the ground while the heel is lifted; however, there is not a lot of weight on the toes.
5. Arms can extend upward, placed on the hips, or another arm variation you enjoy.

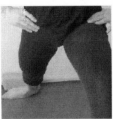

Block against the wall

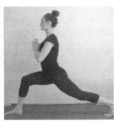

Arms stay low

Modification
• Prop a block against the wall, press back foot into the block.
• If you find it difficult to ground the back heel down to the ground, roll a blanket or a similar prop to place under the back heel until you progress in the pose, you may remove the prop as strength increases.
• Place hands at hips or heart center.
• Back knee rests on a block or other prop, coming into a low or lower lunge.

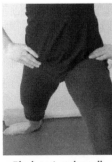

Add a back bend

Deepen
• Raise arms above head, drawing the shoulder blades down.
• Include a back bend, with arms lifted.
• Interlace fingers behind back, opening up the chest and look up.
• Forward fold or incorporate a twist.

Inhale strength, exhale weakness, inhale determination.

WARRIOR I (VIRABHADRASANA I)

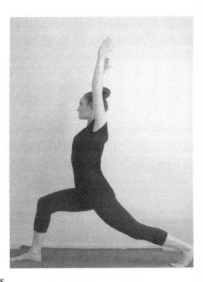

Getting into the Posture
1. From Mountain Pose, step one foot back and rotate the back foot about 45 degrees.
2. Front leg is lunged; knee does not extend past the ankle.
3. Hips face forward, waistline is straight.
4. Extend the arms high while shoulders stay down, biceps near ears.
5. Energetically, the arms are pulling backward (Optional arm variations).

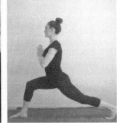

Block against the wall   Arms stay low

Modification
• Prop a block against the wall, press back foot into the block.
• If you find it difficult to ground the back heel down to the ground, roll a blanket or a similar prop to place under the back heel until you progress in the pose, then you may remove the prop.
• Place hands at hips or heart center.

Find your strongest Warrior Pose. Feel the strength of your entire body, especially your legs. Your breath is relaxed, your heart steady. Your negative thoughts are quieted. Inhale "yes" and exhale your "no's." Remember, His strength is perfected in your weakness. You are strong. Root down in Him.

Deepen
• Raise arms above head, drawing the shoulder blades down.
• Include a back bend with arms lifted.
• Interlace fingers behind back, opening up the chest, and look up.
• Forward Fold into Humble Warrior.

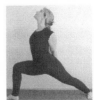

Chest expansion

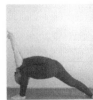

Forward Fold
(Humble Warrior)

WARRIOR II (VIRABHADRASANA II)

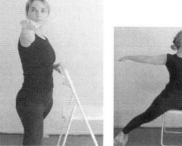

Getting into the Posture
1. From Warrior I, open the hips to the side of the extended leg.
2. Palms come to shoulder height and face down, arms actively engaged.
3. Gaze can be where neck is most comfortable.

Modification
- Prop a block against the wall, press back foot into the block.
- If you find it difficult to ground the back heel down to the ground, roll a blanket or a similar prop to place under the back heel until you progress in the pose, then you may remove the prop.
- Place hands at hips or heart center.
- Look forward instead of over the front fingers.
- Use a chair or bench to rest front thigh upon.
- Hold onto a chair.

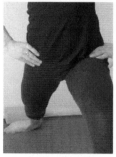 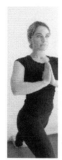 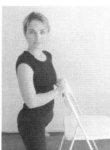 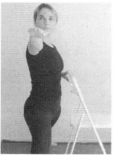 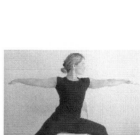

Block against the wall   Keep arms low   Practice with a chair for balance and stability

Deepen
- Rotate inside of the elbows upward, drawing the shoulder blades down.
- Interlace fingers behind back, opening up the chest, and look up.
- Come to Reverse Warrior, sliding the hand (careful to not place weight on leg) down back leg, reaching through the front leg's side body, look up.
- Deepen lunge to cause the front thigh to become parallel to the ground.
- Practice with the hands bound through the legs, someday coming into Bird of Paradise.
- Practice a deep forward fold coming into Humble Warrior.

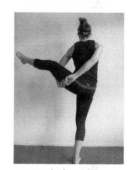

Bird of Paradise

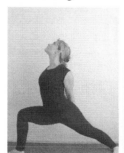 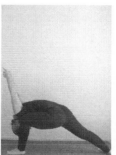 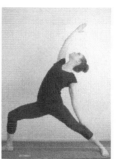

Chest expansion   Humble Warrior   Side/Back bend (Reverse Warrior)

This is time to soar into your deepest expression of this posture. Find balance as you remain rooted to the earth and strong in the mind. Inhale courage in this Warrior stance. Exhale defeat and anything you feel is a weakness. Inhalations bring in composure and contentment.

They helped David against the band of raiders, for they were all mighty men of valor and were commanders in the army. 1 Chronicles 12:21 English Standard Version

HUMBLE WARRIOR / WARRIOR SEAL

He leads the humble in what is right, and teaches the humble His way. Psalm 25:9

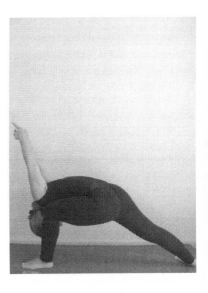

Getting into the Posture

1. From Warrior I, clasp the hands near the lumbar, or the small of the back.
2. Open the heart with a chest expansion by gently pulling the hands down towards the earth.
3. Remain in a strong Warrior stance; nothing in the bottom body will change.
4. Begin to hinge forward with the hips, allowing the arms to come over the head by opening the shoulder blades.
5. Progress into bringing the heart closer to the calf of the front leg.
6. Press through the back edge of the back foot while energetically engaging the inner thighs.
7. Continue to allow the shoulders to open as you gently let your arms come deeper over your head.

Modification

- Prop a block against the wall, press back foot into the block. If you find it difficult to ground the back heel down to the ground, roll a blanket or a similar prop to place under the back heel until you progress in the pose, you may then remove the prop.
- Place hands at hips or heart center.
- Do not hinge; focus on opening and lifting the heart.
- Use the back of a chair, and stay upright.
- Practice Low Lunge or Crescent Lunge.

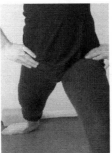 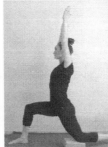 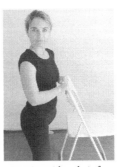

Block against the wall   Add a block   Practice with a chair for balance and stability

Deepen

- Continue to use your breath to work on connecting the forehead to the front leg's shin.
- Deepen the lunge, front thigh parallel to the ground.
- Press the back heel into the ground and engage, lengthen through the entire back leg.
- As tension in the shoulder blade area releases, arms can come further above your head and closer to the ground with each exhale.

Every breath brings in humility. Every exhale sweeps away worry, anxieties, fears and doubts. Continue to release pride, ego, discouragement or wounds from the past and continue to bring in humility. Exhale self-doubt.

REVERSE WARRIOR (VIPARITA VIRABHADRASANA)

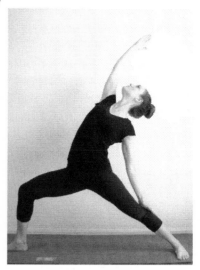

Getting into the Posture

1. From Warrior II, keep the bottom body in a strong Warrior stance (nothing changes in the lower half), using your core muscles, bend the rib cage to the side and backward, towards the straightened leg. Let the back hand "melt down" the leg.
2. Arms reach in opposite directions, breathing into the interior and exterior intercostal muscles.
3. Deepen the lunge of the front leg if possible, eventually the thigh becomes parallel to the earth.

Modification
- Prop a block against the wall, press back foot into the block.
- If you find it difficult to ground the back heel down to the ground, roll a blanket or a similar prop to place under the back heel until you progress in the pose, you may then remove the prop.
- Place hands at hips or heart center.
- Decrease the angle of the back bend.
- Use a chair or wall for support.
- Sit in a chair or on the floor for gentle side bends.
- Straighten front leg.

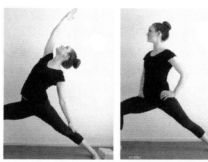

Place block against the wall for stability

Deepen
- Deepen the back bend.
- Increase the lunge, someday getting the front leg's thigh parallel to the ground.
- Press the back heel into the ground and engage, lengthen through the entire back leg.
- Wrap back forearm behind the waist for a bind.
- Bend the top arm and reach behind skull as the elbow reaches toward the sky.

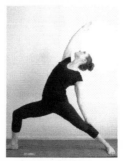

Deepen the back bend

Find your strongest Reverse Warrior and hold it until you realize just how truly strong you are in the Lord. Remember this sensation of true strength and call upon Him next time you are feeling weak, exhausted or less-than.

EXTENDED SIDE ANGLE (UTTHITA PARSVAKONASANA)

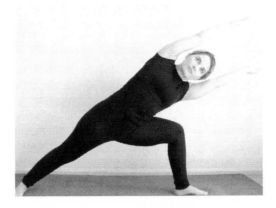

Getting into the Posture

1. From Warrior II, place the front arm to the interior of the lunged foot. You may also rest the forearm on the thigh or place the hand on a block. Wherever the arm or hand is, there is not a lot of weight on it, if you can, use the abdominal to lift the hand off the ground completely.

2. The opposite arm extends upward as your torso leans towards the front lunged leg. Be sure to not cave in or round down. Stay lifted through the core body, keep a long spine, you may also raise both arms as shown.

3. Press through the knife edge of the back foot, deepen the lunge if you are able. Create a long line of energy from the edge of the back foot to the fingertips.

Modification

- Prop a block against the wall, press back foot into the block or press the back heel into the wall directly.
- Place top hand on hip.
- Look forward or down instead of over the front fingers.
- Use a chair or bench to rest front thigh upon until strength is built up.
- Use a block under foundational hand, may be used at the tallest height in the beginning, then on shorter side, then you can remove the block all together as strength is built up.
- Bring hand in front of thigh onto a block or the ground, pressing shoulder into front of bent thigh.

Deepen

- Using core strength, lift through the torso and bring both biceps near your ears as you lengthen through the arms, creating alignment from the back edge of foot to fingertips.
- Using a strap and a 5 to 10 pound weight, loop the strap around front leg and loop through weight. Place the strap around the midline of the thigh, let the weight pull your front leg thigh bone down towards the earth.
- Continue to lengthen throughout the spine, being buoyant in the torso, as you ground through the heels. To lessen, gaze at floor or straight ahead.
- To deepen further gaze is upward.
- Practice with a bind, use a strap if needed.
- Practice Bird of Paradise.

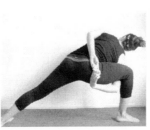

Side Angle with a bind: opens shoulders & chest

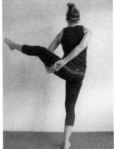

Bird of Paradise

REVOLVED SIDE ANGLE (PARIVRTTA PARSVAKONASANA)

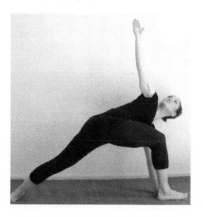

Getting into the Posture

1. From Side Angle, replace the inner hand that is on the earth, with the extended hand.
2. Rotate the torso and reach upward and backward.
3. Pull the navel in towards the spine, let the core do the twisting.
4. Gaze can be upward, forward or down at the ground, whichever is most comfortable on the neck.
5. Try to keep all four corners of both feet rooted to the earth, and continue to press through the knife edge of the back foot engaging the entire leg. It's okay to rotate the back foot and come onto toes to assist in the twist.

Modification

- Lifting the back heel can assist in balancing.
- Prop a block against the wall, press back foot into the block or press the back heel into the wall directly.
- Keep hand placement low and/or foundational hand on a block.
- Look forward or down. Do not turn neck to look upward.
- Keep torso low and forward with no twist.

Remember twists can be as moderate or as intense as you make them. As your spine and surrounding muscles gain flexibility your twists will deepen, causing organs to be even more detoxified (Think of the wash rag being wrung out as you twist). Make sure you are twisting from the abdominal and not using limbs to force the twist, this can torque and injure the back, specifically the lumbar region.

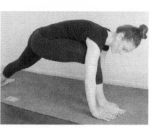

Lessen the twist

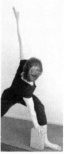

Use a block

Deepen

- All four corners of both feet press into the earth.
- Rotating the back foot will allow a deeper twist.
- Use prayer position and press hands to heart center, one elbow reaching towards the ground, the opposite elbow reaches towards the sky.
- Opening up the arms to reach in opposite direction, lifting through the torso and lengthen through the spine, also allowing for a great chest expansion and heart opener.

TRIANGLE (TRIKONASANA)

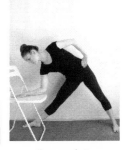

Getting into the Posture
1. From Side Angle, gently take the lunge out of the front leg.
2. Bend the torso over the plane of the front leg.
3. Extend arms in opposite directions, energetically engaging the arms.
4. Keep hips and spine in alignment (Use a block under hand to elevate spine if needed).

Remain buoyant and lifted in the torso. "Lift" the knees and thighs, or engage the leg muscles.

Modification
- Rest top arm on hip.
- Shorten the distance between feet.
- Lift the back heel working up to placing all four corners of both feet on the ground.
- Place the back of the heel or your back against a wall.
- Prop a block against the wall, press back foot into the block or press the back heel into the wall directly.
- Look forward or down instead of at the overhead fingers.
- Use a chair or bench to rest front hand on.
- Use a block or blocks under foundational hand, may be used at the tallest height in the beginning, then on shorter side, then you can remove the block(s) all together as strength is built up.

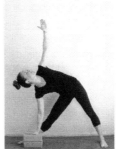 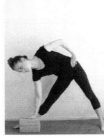 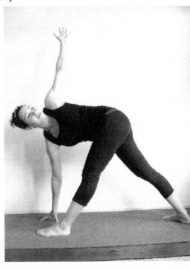

Place block(s) under hand   Gaze and arm stays down   Rest on chair

Deepen
- Front heel is in alignment with the arch of the back foot.
- Staying lifted through the torso, the foundational hand lifts off the block, ground, or leg, radiant in all ten fingers opening and expanding throughout the chest.
- Continue to lift the legs and expand energetically throughout the entire body towards the sky.
- Extend arms, biceps by ears creating a long energetic line from the fingertips to the knife edge of back foot.

To deepen further come into…

REVOLVED TRIANGLE POSE (PARIVRTTA TRIKONASANA)

Getting into the Posture
1. From Triangle, bring the top arm to the inside of the front foot (Or the exterior of the foot for more of a challenge, attempt to get fingers and toes flush).
2. Using the core muscles, gently rotate the torso inward.
3. Extend the hand that was to the interior of the foot back and upward. Energetically engaging the arms and keeping alignment from wrist to wrist (Use a block under the hand on the ground to elevate spine if needed).
5. Remain buoyant and lifted in the torso.
6. Lift the knees and thighs.
7. Draw the navel in towards the spine.

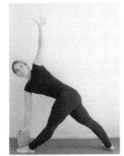

Modified Reverse Triangle

Inhale clarity and strength, exhale confusion. Set your mind to stay in this posture and feel the vitality and fortitude of your mind, body and spirit. Breathe in, "I am strong in the Lord."

Each inhalation brings in intuition and discernment, every exhalation rids the body of confusion. Focus on strength, balance, clarity and every fiber of your body being at ease as you settle into this posture, know that everything is going to be okay as you inhale reassurance.

Jesus said to her, "I am the resurrection and the life.
Whoever believes in Me, though he die, yet shall he live. John 11:25

STANDING POSTURES
CHAIR POSE (UTKATASANA)

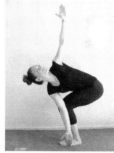

Getting into the Posture
1. From Mountain Pose, feet together or hip width, deeply bend both knees as if you are sitting back into a chair.
2. Hollow out the belly (Pull the navel in towards the spine).
3. Look down and make sure you can see your toes, if you cannot, sit back further.
4. Hands can be at hips, heart center or biceps near ears.
(You may find more stability with your feet together, if so, engage the ankles, knees and thighs together)

Modifications
- Keep hands by side, on hips or at heart center.
- Sit on edge of chair, lengthen spine, perhaps add a forward fold.
- Use a wall for support, perhaps placing a block in between thighs and engage inner thighs.

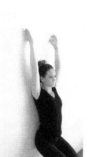 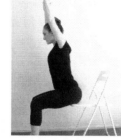 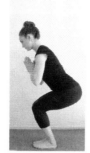

Stand against wall   Use chair   Hands to heart or hips

Deepen
- Raise arms above head.
- Close your eyes.
- Incorporate a twist from the torso side to side.
- Use a block or book to squeeze in between the inner thighs, helping to further strengthen the thighs.
- Come to balls of the feet and sit back further, arms extend in front of you with palms facing down or inward, be sure to create space between the shoulders and ears.
- Move with each breath (Vinyasa), squatting and/or twisting.

To further explore, from chair practice…

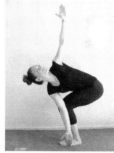

Add a twist

SIDE CROW (PARSVA BAKASANA)

Getting into the Posture
1. From Revolved Chair, bend the knees into a deep squat so the heels and buttocks connect.
2. Deeply twist bringing the arms to one side as the triceps connect with outer thighs.
3. Slightly bend the elbows to create a "shelf" for the triceps, the feet and knees continue to face forward.
4. As you exhale, hinge the torso toward the earth as you lift your toes off the ground. Breathe. Settle in.

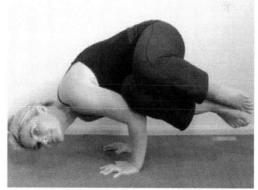

    This posture is about mind over body. Inhale tenacity. You will need to rely on, and inhale His might and power, as you exhale your own weaknesses and powerlessness. Steady your heart and calm your thoughts. In Him, you are strong. Fierce. Unstoppable. Let that settle into your spirit as you sink down closer to the earth.

INTENSE SIDE STRETCH (PARSVOTTANASANA)

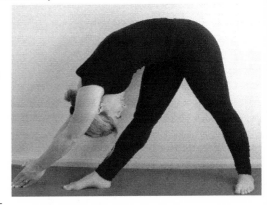

Getting into the Posture

1. From Upward Salute, bring hands to Prayer Salutation, step one foot back, toes of back foot turn slightly outward.
2. Keeping both legs straightened as much as possible without locking the knees, hips squared to front, hinge at the hips into a forward fold.
3. Choose arm variation. Keep prayer salutation or bring hands to floor, walk them back to the midline of the body, experiment and choose the variation that works for you.
4. In the forward fold, root all four corners of both feet firmly into the earth.
5. Lift both hamstrings and thighs energetically towards the sky.
6. Allow the head to hang heavy, full expression tucks the chin in towards the chest gazing at the navel, forehead to knee. You may bend the front leg to assist in the knee-forehead connection until greater flexibility is achieved.

Modification

- Prop a block against the wall, press back foot into the block. If you find it difficult to ground the back heel down to the ground, roll a blanket or a similar prop to place under the back heel until you progress in the pose, eventually remove the prop.
- Keep spine elevated by placing hands on blocks (Begin with tallest height until flexibility increases). May also use the seat or back of a chair.
- Micro-bend both knees or one knee, working up to lengthening through both legs as your breath assists you in straightening out the knees someday. The full benefit of intense side stretch is to eventually have both legs straightened, without hyper extending the knee, and all four corners of both feet rooted down.

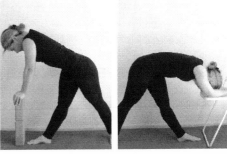

Use as many props as necessary in any posture.

Deepen

- Continue to use your breath to work on connecting the forehead to the front leg's shin.
- Tuck chin in towards the chest, gazing at the naval, which massages the thyroid and parathyroid gland to increase metabolism.
- Press all four corners of both feet into the earth as you lift both thighs towards the sky.
- Practice Standing Splits.

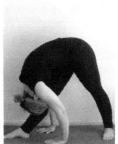

Hands to mid line   Standing Splits

Each inhalation brings in His energy, stability and life force. Every exhalation brings your heart and limbs closer together as you squeeze out weakness, toxins and "self". Focus on new breath and life as you create space by getting rid of things that your body and you no longer need. You will physically, emotionally, mentally and spiritually be making room for invincibility, intrepidity and boldness in the Lord, create space for the Lord to work in your life! Allow your doubts, worries and anxieties to disappear so that He may speak to you here.

Prayer:
Father, thank You for strengthening me and reviving my soul with energy to face each day and any trial. I praise You that You have created me to do Your will and that You have it all worked out and I don't have to worry about anything! Nothing I have gone through will be wasted. Psalm 138:8 says that You are perfecting everything that concerns me, You even prosper my mistakes! I come to You now in all humility and surrender everything to You, my strength, my mind, my spirit, my soul, all my emotions and all of my relationships. I ask that You take it all and conform these to Your will. Thank You for taking my messes and causing them to be messages that will draw others to You. Have Your way in my life today Lord. I stand firm, immovable, and rooted in your promises.
With all that I have I praise You! Amen and Amen!

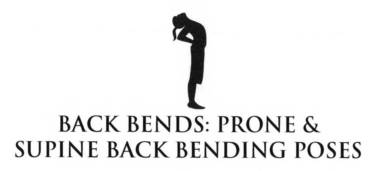

BACK BENDS: PRONE & SUPINE BACK BENDING POSES

To You, Lord, I have lifted up my soul. Psalm 25:1

Throughout the Bible we see the importance of our prayer postures. Prone or prostate postures are portrayed as an urgent cry or plea to the Lord out of desperation. Bowing down on our knees, we read, is an act of humility and surrender. Standing prayers are seen as praise and worship, giving thanks to the Lord. Back bends will not only be a posture of praise and worship, but also an incredible way to lift your heart and soul to the Lord. Most prone postures are back bends, so you may use these postures for a plea to the Lord as well as an offering of praise.

If only you would prepare your heart and lift up your hands to Him in prayer! Job 11:13

Do you ever wake up in the morning grateful just to be alive? Does your heart get overwhelmed at the many blessings you have? Maybe it is as simple as the breath in your body. You know, some people no longer have this simple pleasure. Perhaps it is as simple as having a car that gets you from point "A" to "B." Some days, I wake up and just want to thank the Lord for waking me up. A standing back bend can help us pause, stand firm, lift our hearts and praise our Heavenly Father.

Because these poses come from leg strength, the bottom half of your body must be completely engaged for a successful back bend. As we talked about in the standing postures, you have to root down in the feet. Be strong in the Lord, and then you can rise up and lift your heart towards the heavens.

It was strong and beautiful, with wide-spreading branches, for its roots went deep into abundant water.
Ezekiel 31:7 New Living Translation

As with twists, you can incorporate back bend poses into many postures, including seated, standing, balancing, prone or supine poses. The nervous, digestive and metabolic systems are all stimulated in back-bending postures. These postures are known to be rejuvenating and invigorating. For this reason, it may not be a good idea to practice them near bedtime. Back bends stretch and release the chest muscles, allowing circulation to flow freely to the heart and lungs. Mental clarity and focus can be a result of back bends as cerebral spinal fluids are circulated throughout the system. Back bends also stimulate the lymphatic system, pumping lymphatic fluids by opening the chest, armpits and groin areas where lymph nodes and glands are located. Back bends cause pressure on the kidneys and adrenals, which not only enhances the cleansing action, but also releases adrenaline, causing an invigorating sensation while stimulating your metabolism.

In any back bend, be reminded of your prayer and praise posture. You may feel like you've gone jogging after a back bend; allow that energy and fresh oxygen to flow throughout your body. Always release any back bend gently and rest a moment if needed.

The Lord is my strength and my shield. My heart trusted Him, so I received help. My heart is triumphant;
I give thanks to Him with my song. Psalm 28:7

In a back-bending posture, the spine remains pliable. Strength is required and developed throughout the entire body. Back bends are dynamic postures that move to counter gravity. These postures need to be incorporated for a well-balanced practice as they will stretch and strengthen the front of the abdomen, hips, thighs, shoulders, spine and chest. A lot of stress, tension or trauma can be trapped in our core centers. These postures can help release deep tension, mild depression and emotional trauma. Both twists and back bends will not only cleanse and rejuvenate, but will also leave you with a calm balance and an overall sense of well-being.

It is always a good idea to release the worked muscles from back bends by doing forward folds, being careful to release the sacrum safely and effectively by not moving from one extreme to the other. An example is an intense standing back bend, immediately into a deep forward fold. Stop at a halfway point and allow the sacrum to release. When you feel it release, continue. Individuals with serious back injuries and women who are pregnant or menstruating should, in general, avoid deep back bends.

Remember that a successful back bend comes from the strength of the legs. By engaging our legs we protect the spine as we strengthen the entire backside. Generally speaking, we spend a lot of time strengthening the front side of our body; it takes time to build up the strength of our typically weaker backside. The other important thing to remember is to breathe. It is very easy to hold your breath in back bends as the vocal cords and throat become constricted, but this is a good thing and provides many benefits to the neck and throat. Although your breath is constricted (sometimes greatly), take "sips of air" instead of holding your breath. Hold the pose, not the breath. Always remember to have patience with any asana or asana family. The more that you practice the better you will become.

Benefits of back bends include, but are not limited to:
- Strengthens back muscles, arms, shoulders, neck, throat, thighs and buttocks.
- Improves alignment of the spine.
- Improves posture and increases mobility of spine.
- Stretches the entire front body, specifically feet, ankles, thighs, groin and hip flexors.
- Stretches and opens the neck, chest, lungs, shoulders, side bodies and abdominal area.
- Strengthens the respiratory, cardiovascular, lymphatic and endocrine systems.
- Stretches throat, thyroid, and parathyroid glands, stimulating metabolism.
- Stimulates digestion and aids in circulation.
- Can be therapeutic for mild cases of sciatica, asthma and osteoporosis.
- Therapeutic for flat feet, backaches and indigestion.
- Can relieve constipation, menstrual discomfort and menopause symptoms.
- Relieves stress, anxiety and depression.
- Increases stamina, energizes and rejuvenates.
- Improves concentration, balance, focus, coordination, mental clarity and memory.
- Invigorating, energizing and renewing.

Cautions include, but are not limited to:
- Those with severe sciatica, asthma, arthritis, insomnia, vertigo or glaucoma.
- Those with headache or migraine, severe back, shoulder, hip and neck injury or pregnancy (specifically second and third trimester).

DIG INTO THE WORD. YOUR SOUL WORK; ISAIAH 57:12-15 A MEDITATION FOR BACK BENDS

THE POSTURES

STANDING BACK BEND (ANUVITTASANA)

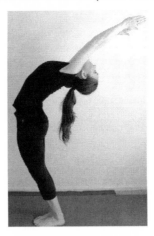

Getting into the Posture

1. From Mountain pose, inhale as you extend your arms overhead, biceps near ears.

Options: Palms can come together as arms are lifted, or a modification is to place your fingertips facing downward on the tailbone area for assistance. Pull your elbows in and back.

2. Engage the legs as you root your feet down into the earth.

3. Using your leg and core strength, gently press the pelvic and core body forward.

4. Taking small sips of air, but not holding your breath, let your throat and upper back open and release back; allow the head to "hang heavy" (unless you have serious neck and spine issues).

5. When you are ready to release your back bend, gently come out of the posture into upward salute, then fold half way forward, after sacrum releases, exhale into a full Standing Forward Fold.

     Allow your body, spine and sacrum to gently release instead of going from one extreme of a back bend to the other extreme of a deep forward fold. This will ensure safety and cause no shock to your systems.

Modification

- Lessen the back bend.
- Practice Cat-Cow or Cat-Cow Seated.
- Do not extend arms above head.
- Place fists or hands (fingertips facing upward towards the sky) on the small of the back to assist in a slightly deeper back bend. If you choose this modification, abduct your shoulder blades, and bring your elbows to face backward, opening up the chest, heart and lungs.
- Hands can also come to heart center (Prayer/Anjali Mudra).
- Clasp hands at the small of your back, and focus on lifting your heart instead of deepening the back bend.
- Stand with back facing a wall, place hands on the wall at your level of choice above the head, waist level, etc., and use the wall to assist with the back bend.

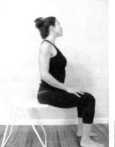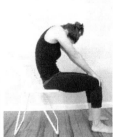

Cat-Cow seated, mild or deep back bend

Deepen

- Increase back bend.
- Gaze back or at the floor. Continue to focus the shoulder blades away from the ears, lifting heart center towards the sky. If you have a neck injury, avoid this. Inhale to lengthen from the spine. As you and exhale, find depth.
- Clasp hands at the small of your back and deepen the back bend.
- Walk hands down the back of legs; work down to Wheel Pose.
- Add a sequence; from Standing to Wheel back to Standing.

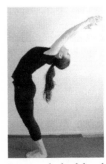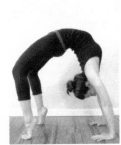

Increase the back bend   Practice Wheel

LORD OF THE DANCE POSE (NATARAJASANA)

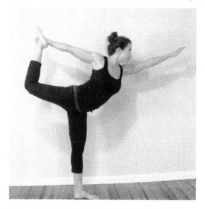

Getting into the Posture

1. From Mountain Pose, bend one knee, with heel as close to the buttocks as possible. Clasp the same hand (a variation can be the opposite hand reaches for the interior of this foot) to the inner foot or the first toes. You may also reach further up the leg or shin for this posture.
2. Bring the knee back into alignment and draw it near the other knee.
3. As you inhale, extend the opposite arm towards the sky and find length in the body.
4. As you exhale, energetically kick into the hand creating space between the glute and heel.
5. Begin to hinge from the hips, bringing the bent leg's thigh parallel with the earth.
6. The opposite extended arm comes forward or upward depending on the variation, palm facing out or down, energetically kicking, reaching and stretching in opposite directions.

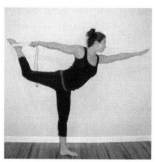

Practice with strap and/or wall

Modification

- Use a strap around ankle.
- Place one hand on a chair or wall until you achieve balance and strength.

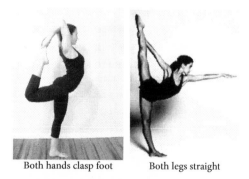

Both hands clasp foot   Both legs straight

Deepen

- Opposite hand to foot, reach for the inside of the foot, using your breath to increase the back bend as you focus on lifting the heart towards the sky.
- Reach closer up the leg towards the knee, straightening out the extended leg.
- Both hands grab the extended foot or leg.
- Practice Standing Splits, both legs straighten.

BACK BENDING POSTURES
CAT-COW (BITILASANA)

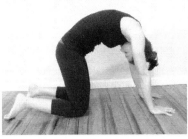
Cat

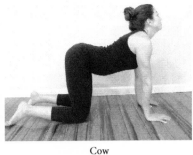
Cow

Getting into the Posture

1. From Child's Pose, come into a Table Top position, shoulders above the wrists and hips above the knees. Knees are separated, hip-width apart.
2. With inhalations, drop your belly as you exaggerate lifting the tailbone and gaze to the sky (Cow).
3. As you exhale, tuck your sacrum under as you draw your navel up and into your spine, simultaneously tucking your chin into your chest. Draw your shoulder blades apart. Everything "tucks in" for Cat.
4. Enjoy flowing in and out of Cat-Cow with the breath, or hold one posture and enjoy more breaths in each posture.
5. Option as you transition: bend the elbows to engage the chest as you flow.

Modification

- Lessen the back bend.
- Do not gaze upward.
- Use a blanket under your knees.
- Practice flowing or static postures sitting on the edge of a chair.
- Cat-Cow seated postures.

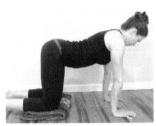 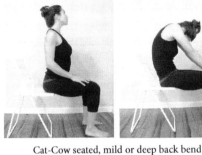 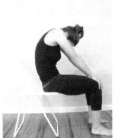

Place blanket under knees

Cat-Cow seated, mild or deep back bend

Deepen

- Increase back bend.
- Micro-bend elbows as you flow into each posture, engaging more of the chest region.
- Inhale to lengthen (from neutral spine position) the opposite hand and leg. As you exhale, tuck the elbow and knee close into each other as you tuck your chin into your chest. Repeat as many times as desired and switch to other side.
- Energetically press your heel back and reach your fingertips forward. Your core is completely engaged and you want to feel the sensation of someone "pulling" you in opposite directions. Imagine someone gently pulling your wrist and another person gently pulling your opposite ankle that is lifted.

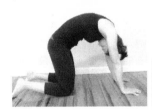 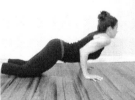 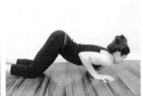 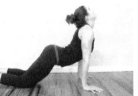 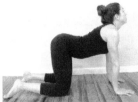

Flowing through Cat-Cow keeps a micro bend in the elbows

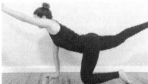 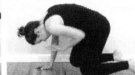 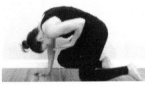

Add arm balance and a knee crunch for a strengthening

Continue to focus the shoulder blades away from the ears, lifting heart center towards the sky. If you have a neck injury, avoid this. Exaggerate pulling the navel back towards the spine. This will greatly improve your posture and strengthen the core and wrists.

To further deepen this posture, extend leg back and reach opposite hand out for...

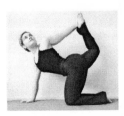

TIGER / STRETCHING TIGER (VYAGHRASANA)

Pronated Back Bends

Pronated postures (belly down) stretch and increase flexibility in the entire back, specifically the lower back, while strengthening the muscles of the chest, shoulders, arms, legs and abdomen. These postures also tone the nerves, extensors and muscles in the neck and shoulder areas. The majority of prone poses are back bends, which energize the entire body, toning and massaging abdominal organs, specifically the kidneys, therefore improving digestion, blood circulation and stimulating the reproductive organs. Prone postures can reduce fatigue and stress as well as help people with respiratory disorders such as asthma.

Prone postures can be easy enough for beginners as well as challenging as a practitioner builds up to holding postures for long periods or adding strengthening moves and flows. Prone postures should be avoided if a headache or migraine is present. Also avoid if you have high or low blood pressure, a hernia, neck injury, pain in the lower back or a recent abdominal surgery. Women should avoid practicing deep back-bending postures during pregnancy.

Remember, in scripture, pronated postures symbolize an urgent request or standing in the gap for intercessory.

Dig into the Word. Your Soul Work; Psalm 139
A Meditation on Pronated Back Bends

PRONATED BACK BENDS

SPHINX (SALAMBA BHUJANGASANA)

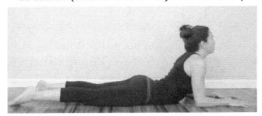

Getting into the Posture

1. From a prone position, place your elbows under your shoulders so that your forearms are parallel and resting on the floor.
2. Engage the legs as you actively press the toes down and out towards the back.
3. Energetically draw the tailbone down towards the feet; legs are active and face is relaxed.
4. As you inhale, lift the torso into this mild back bend. Use the belly to soften the lower back, energetically widening the sacrum region.
5. Shoulder blades are back and down, away from the ears.
6. Buttocks are engaged, but not clinched.
7. Taking 5 to 10 breaths in Sphinx, gently come out of it and rest one cheek on the ground. Repeat if desired.

Modification

- Lessen the back bend.
- Use blanket or other prop under arms, sternum, pelvis, and/or under thighs.
- Neck injury keeps the head level, also known as a neutral gaze.
- Place forearms on a wall standing up.
- Practice Crocodile (Makarasana) by itself as a resting pose or between other prone back bends. Elbows slide forward, above the shoulders and forehead rests on forearms. Legs are further than hip-width apart; toes point outward and rest on the interior of the foot.

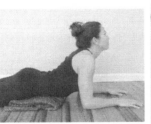
Use blanket or bolster

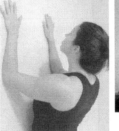
Practice with wall

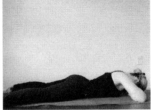
Crocodile Pose

Deepen

- Increase back bend.
- Continue to focus the shoulder blades away from the ears, lifting heart center towards the sky (Neck injury keeps gaze neutral or on ground).
- Use exhalation to deepen the back bend.
- You may also flow with your breath into Dolphin pose (Ardha Pincha Mayurasana). Keeping forearms on the earth, lift tailbone into Dolphin and come back into Sphinx for a full body strengthener.
- Practice Cobra or Upward-Facing Dog.

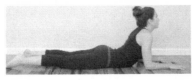
Inhale Sphinx

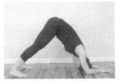
Exhale Dolphin

BACK BENDING POSTURES
LOCUST (SALABHASANA)

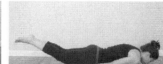

Getting into the Posture

1. From a prone position, place your chin on your mat, and "kiss the ground." You may want to cushion your pelvis and/or ribs with a blanket.
2. Place palms in front of the hips, planted on the earth as if you were setting up to hit a volleyball, exterior of pinky fingers may touch, or clasp fingers together.
3. Turning your thighs inward, activate your legs and firm the buttocks.
4. On an inhale, lift the lower body upward.
5. Gently release everything down to the earth.
6. Allow gravity to help you release and "melt" everything down. You may gently bend your knees here and "windshield-wiper" them to release the pose further.

Modification

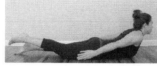 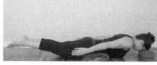

Lessen the back bend, lower the legs   Blanket and block(s) to support and assist

- Lessen the back bend, or practice Sphinx or Crocodile.
- Use a blanket or other prop under sternum, pelvis, forehead, and/or under thighs.
- Rest forehead on a block or rolled blanket.
- Keep hands on floor.
- Alternate lifting one foot at a time instead of both.
- Use a rolled blanket under your arms.
- Lift only the legs or only the torso instead of both at the same time.

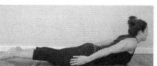 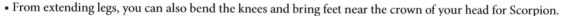

Practice one leg at a time   Feet and knees together, palms facing forward

Deepen

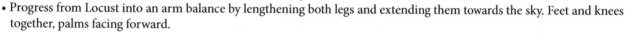

- Increase back bend.
- Continue to focus the shoulder blades back and downward, lifting heart center towards the sky. Neck injury keeps gaze neutral or on ground.
- Use exhalation to deepen the back bend.
- Extend arms and legs, "swim" opposite leg and extended arm "paddle."
- Place hands behind head, elbows out wide, moving slowly up and down for another strengthening move.
- A deeper expression of Locust is to bend the legs, bring knees together. With each inhale, the torso, arms, and legs lift as you focus on lifting the knees further away from the earth with each breath.
- Progress from Locust into an arm balance by lengthening both legs and extending them towards the sky. Feet and knees together, palms facing forward.
- From extending legs, you can also bend the knees and bring feet near the crown of your head for Scorpion.

Scorpion

COBRA (BHUJANGASANA)

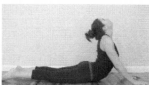

Getting into the Posture

1. From a prone position, bend your elbows and bring them tightly into the rib cage, much like grasshopper wings, fingertips underneath the shoulders.
2. Press the tops of the feet into the earth; allow your inhalations to lift you off the earth.
3. Keep a micro-bend in the elbows as you draw your shoulder blades back and down.
4. Lift your heart and collarbone towards the sky.
5. If the neck allows, release your gaze to the sky.
6. Holding for up to 30 seconds, gently releasing, place one cheek to the floor and rest.

Modification

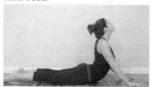 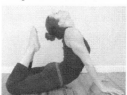

Gaze upward   Deepen the back bend

- Lessen the back bend; do not come up as far.
- Practice Sphinx or Baby Cobra.
- Use blanket or other prop under sternum and/or pelvis.

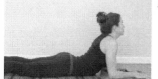

Practice Sphinx

Deepen

- Increase back bend by walking hands closer towards the chest; straighten arms without locking the elbows.
- Continue to focus the shoulder blades back and downward, away from the ears, lifting heart center towards the sky.
- Use exhalation to deepen the back bend.
- Bend the knees, practice Extended / King Cobra (Raja Bhujangasana).

Extended Cobra

BACK BENDING POSTURES
UPWARD FACING DOG (URDHVA MUKHA SVANASANA)

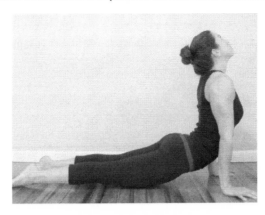

Getting into the Posture

1. From a prone posture (may also come from Downward-Facing Dog), place the palms near your waistline and spread all ten fingers out wide; elbows "hug" the rib cage.
2. Press the tops of both feet into the earth as you engage the legs and firm the buttocks.
3. As you inhale, press firmly into the earth as you lift your torso and legs off the ground.
4. Arms straighten out as the inner elbows face inward and your hands are energetically pulling back. Upward Facing Dog is considered an arm balance, so think of your hands and fingers as "feet and toes" here.
5. Shoulder blades roll back and down, away from your ears.
6. You may hold this posture, use it in a sequence, "Son" Salutation or simply come back to a prone posture. Place one cheek down and rest arms by your side relaxing the entire body.

Let us return to the Lord. We lift up our heart and hands toward God in heaven. Lamentations 3:40-41

Modification
- Lessen the back bend.
- Use a blanket or other prop under sternum and/or pelvis.
- Keep thighs on earth.
- Practice Cobra, Locust or Sphinx.

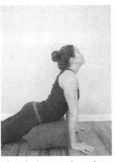

Place bolster under pelvis

Deepen
- Increase back bend by walking hands closer towards the chest; straighten arms without locking the elbows.
- Continue to focus the shoulder blades away from the ears, lifting heart center towards the sky.
- Use exhalation to deepen the back bend.
- Press heels back as you lift hamstrings towards the sky.

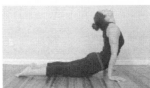

Deepen back bend and gaze

BACK BENDING POSTURES
BOW POSE (DHANURASANA)

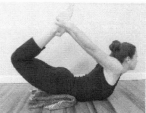

Getting into the Posture

1. Coming from Locust, bend your knees and clasp around the ankles, feet or shins with both hands. Try not to let the knees separate too much; bring them inwardly about hip-width apart or slightly greater than hip-width apart.
2. Gaze at floor. As you inhale, kick into the hands, allowing the thighs to lift off the ground.
3. Open up the heart and chest, allowing the collarbone to lift, or "smile," upward.
4. Only gaze up towards the sky if the neck allows.
5. Continue to kick energetically into the hands, the heels actively kicking away from the buttocks, eventually establishing a raindrop shape in your deepest expression.
6. Hold up to 30 seconds or longer.

Modification

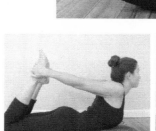
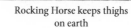

Rocking Horse keeps thighs on earth   Assisted Bow

- Lessen the back bend.
- Practice Cobra or Locust Pose.
- Use strap around ankles or blanket under thighs or sternum.
- Keep thighs on ground (Rocking Horse). You may use a strap around the ankles and focus only on opening up the heart and chest.
- Do not grab hold of feet, only lift upward and breathe.
- Only practice on one side at a time, one leg at a time.

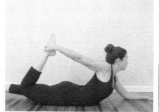
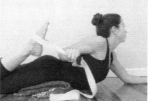
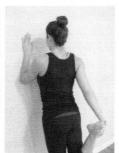
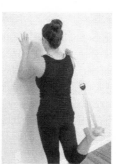

One Legged Bow   One leg with strap   Use a wall   Wall and strap

Deepen

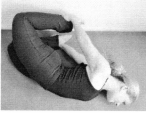

- Increase back bend.
- Calves, thighs and inner feet touch, using the breath continue to work on feet and head someday connecting.
- Roll onto one shoulder and come into Side Bow (Parsva Dhanurasana), using breath to increase back bend and "kicking" into hands for a wonderful chest expansion.

Side Bow

To further deepen Bow Pose, practice...

ADVANCED BOW (PADANGUSTHA DHANURASANA)

Advanced Bow further tones the core, spine and works the shoulders deeply.

Getting into the Posture

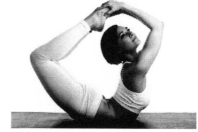

1. From Bow, clasp one foot at a time, reaching for the toes.
2. Grab the other toes; elbows will rotate outward and upward as you clasp the top of the feet.
3. One day the arms straighten as the curve in the lower back is increased.

Steady your breath, heart and thoughts. Listen carefully to the sound of your heartbeat. Realize that means purpose! Your heart is beating because you have purpose here on planet Earth. Feel your strength in this posture. Lifting your heart and settle into the truth that you are strong. Exhale weakness. Inhale strength.

The Lord is my strength and my shield; my heart trusts in Him, and He helps me. My heart leaps for joy, and with my song I praise Him. Psalm 28:7

To further deepen, practice...

FROG POSE (BHEKASANA)

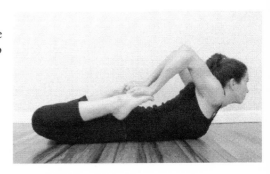

Getting into the Posture
1. From a prone position bend one leg; reach the same side hand to the interior of the foot. Internally rotating the elbow inward, allow the palm of the hand to press the top of the foot down towards the earth.
2. Straighten out the opposite arm, keeping the torso and hips squared to the front (Half Frog).
3. Bend the other leg, internally rotating that elbow to the interior of the inner foot and pressing the palm down on the front of the foot in towards the earth.
4. Lift the torso and heart upward while stretching the front side of the body out (Frog).
5. Gently releasing, extend legs, rest arms by sides and one cheek on the ground.

Modify by practicing Half Frog (Ardha Bhekasana), come to forearm or use a blanket where needed.

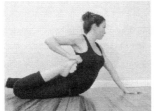
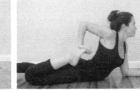
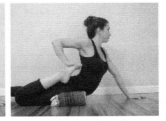

Half Frog   Come to forearm   Place blanket under pelvis

GHERANDA POSE (SUKHA GHERANDASANA)

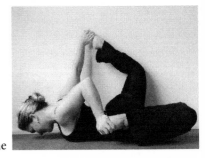

Gheranda Pose is a combination of Bow and Frog Pose. It increases the stretch to the quadriceps, further massaging internal organs and toning the abdominal region.

Getting into the Posture
1. From Half Frog, bring the other leg into Half Bow, eventually straightening leg.

To practice another variation of Frog, start in Sphinx and gently slide your tailbone upward as the knees come apart, beyond the hips. Allow the forearms to settle into the earth, pull the navel in towards the spine and breathe into the hips.

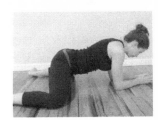

Modification
- Use a bolster, pillow or similar prop under lower ribs to lift torso upward.
- Stay in Half Frog, using one arm or forearm to assist with upper body weight.
- Stand with one hand on wall or chair; bring your ankle into the opposite hand and stretch the front of the thigh. Switch sides. Use a strap around the ankle if needed.

Deepen
- Increase back bend by walking hands closer towards the chest.
- Let the pelvis gently melt toward the earth.

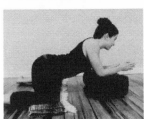

Bolster and blanket

He fell with His face to the ground and prayed, "My Father, if it is possible, may this cup be taken from me. Yet not as I will, but as You will." Matthew 26:39

SUPINE BACK BENDS

BRIDGE (SETU BANDHA SARVANGASANA)

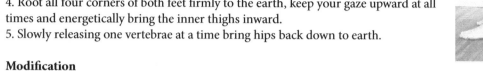

Getting into the Posture

1. From a supine position, bend the knees and bring the soles of the feet towards the tailbone, keeping the feet underneath the knees.
2. As you inhale, lift the hips off the ground, keeping knees and feet hip-width apart and facing forward.
3. Open up the chest and shoulders by walking the shoulder blades back and down, perhaps clasping the hands together, or clasping each ankle.
4. Root all four corners of both feet firmly to the earth, keep your gaze upward at all times and energetically bring the inner thighs inward.
5. Slowly releasing one vertebrae at a time bring hips back down to earth.

Modification

- Place a blanket under the shoulders and/or under the head.
- Use strap around ankles, focusing on lifting the collar bone towards the sky.
- Use a block/blanket/bolster under sacrum and rest the pelvis on support.
- Use a large pillow vertically along the spine and practice a restorative Bridge.
- Use bolster and a blanket under the head.

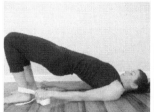
Strap around ankles

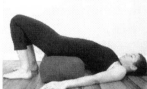
Bolster lifts hips

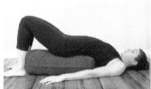
Bolster lifts hips and
stretches abdominal

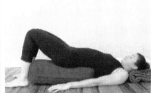
Practice with bolster and blanket

Deepen

- Lift heels off the floor and push your tailbone up.
- Calves, thighs and inner feet touch.
- Extend one leg up; hold for up to a minute.
- Practice with one leg extended or Pigeon legs (cross one ankle over opposite knee), inhaling hips upward, exhaling and slowly lowering for a power move. Repeat 8-12 times on one side and change sides.
- Place a block or book between thighs to engage inner thighs and glutes.

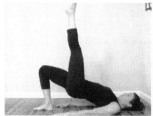
One Legged Bridge

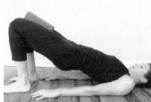
Squeeze the block

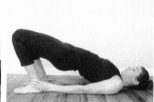
Grab for ankles

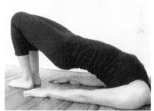
Ankles, knees, thighs together

To deepen this posture you may also practice another Bridge Variation...

BRIDGE POSTURE (SETU BANDHASANA)

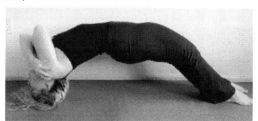

Getting into the Posture

1. For the advanced practitioner only: From a supine posture, bring the heels approximately two feet from glutes.
2. The feet point outwardly about 45 degrees as the heels touch, knees are out wide. Like Fish, the inhalations will lift your chest upwardly as you arch your back greatly.
3. Palms come to ears, fingertips face the shoulders (like Wheel Prep).
4. Lift the hips as much as possible while you balance on the crown of the head and feet. Simultaneously, straighten the legs as you rest on the crown as shown, roll onto the forehead or the whole face to floor. Last expression is crossing the arms to rest each hand on the opposite shoulder.

BACK BENDING POSTURES
CAMEL POSE (USTRASANA)

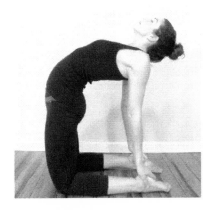

Getting into the Posture

1. Kneeling, with both knees about hip-width apart, bring your thighs perpendicular to the earth. Press the shins and tops of feet into the ground. Buttocks are firm, not clinched.
2. Press the palms to the base of the buttocks, with fingers facing down as you pull the elbows back.
3. Pressing the pelvis forward, maintain the thighs as perpendicular.
4. Progressing, slightly turn the torso one way as you place one hand on the heel of a foot and respectively on the other side. If this is difficult, come to the toes and elevate the heels, allowing your hands and heels to connect more easily. Bring pelvis center and deepen your back bend.
5. Gaze where neck is comfortable. Allow your throat to open but keep it softened. If there are no neck issues, allow the head to hang heavy.
6. Release Camel with caution, stopping when torso is straight, gently lower down to Table Top into mild Cat-Cows or gently make your way into a Child's Pose.

Modification

- Use a wall to support the top of your head (soles of feet press against wall). Protecting the neck, hands press against wall or support pelvis.
- Come to toes, elevating the heels.
- Use the seat of a chair or bench to rest hands or elbows behind you on the seat.
- Use blocks at their tallest height on the exterior of both ankles.

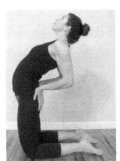
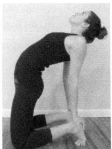
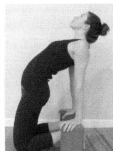
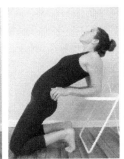
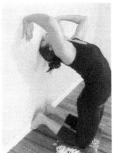

Hands on small of back   Lift toes   Blocks at tallest height   Lean back on seat   Use a wall and blanket

Deepen

- Calves, thighs and inner feet touch, and/or head rests on floor, lifting through pelvis (King Pigeon).
- Recline onto the back and reach for opposite elbows above head.
- If upright, increase the back bend by pressing the tops of the feet into the earth with both hands.
- Continue to use your breath to lift the heart towards the sky, allowing the head to hang heavy.

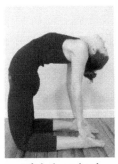

Lift the heart, head
is heavy

Continue to deepen by practicing…

KING PIGEON POSTURE (KAPOTASANA)

Getting into the Posture

1. From Camel, walk your hands further behind you, placing palms on floor, fingers face the feet.
2. Allow the chest to open and lift upward.
3. Gently bend the elbows and come to the forearms, hands to clasp the feet or back of knees someday.
4. Lift the heart, head is heavy.
5. Lightly rest on the crown of the head.

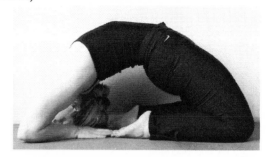

UPWARD BOW / WHEEL (URDHVA DHANURASANA)

Getting into the Posture

1. From a supine position, bring your heels toward the tailbone.
2. Bring your palms near your head; spread all ten fingers out facing the shoulders, palms rooted to the earth.
3. Keep knees hip-width apart, feet firmly planted.
4. Press palms into the earth as you lift your hips up, pausing on the top of the crown.
5. On an inhale, simultaneously press hands and feet into the ground as you straighten your arms, lifting your heart.
6. Buttocks are firm. Let your head hang heavy, or look towards the floor.
7. Stay in your deepest expression of your wheel for 20-30 seconds.
8. Slowly release the posture the same way you got into the pose.
9. Gently come to the crown of your head, pausing and then slowly come all the way down to the ground.
10. Bring your knees into the chest and give yourself a gentle hug.

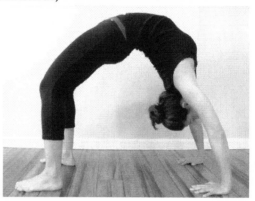

Modification

- Use blocks against the wall and/or on top of a non-stick mat, under hands and/or feet.
- Remain in Bridge until shoulders open and strength is gained.
- Use an exercise ball, ottoman or the seat of a chair to drape your self over.

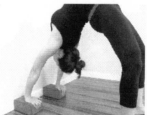

Place blocks against wall   Drape over furniture

Deepen

- Walk hands and feet closer together.
- Press your tailbone toward the ceiling.
- Press forearms into the floor or extend one leg, holding up to 30 seconds, or both simultaneously.
- Practice Wheel or a variation of Wheel.

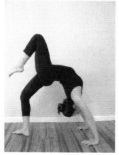 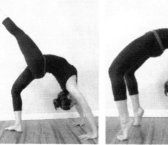 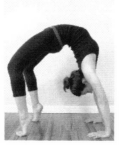 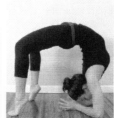

One Legged Wheel   Walk limbs closer together   Come to forearms

Continue to...

UPWARD FACING TWO-LEGGED INVERTED STAFF POSE (DWI PADA VIPARITA DANDASANA)

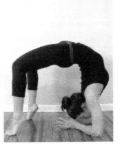

Getting into the Posture

1. From Wheel, bring your palms near your head; spread all ten fingers out facing the shoulders, palms are rooted.
2. Keep knees hip-width apart and feet firmly planted.
3. Bring your elbows and forearms to the earth as you gently come to the crown of your head.
4. Slowly walk one hand at a time behind the skull, interlacing all ten fingers.
5. Press the inner elbows strongly into the ground as you lift your chest and head off the earth.
6. Lift the core body upward. Gently begin to walk one leg out at a time, extending both legs straight with feet on the ground. Press the inner foot into the earth.
7. Holding this posture 20 to 30 seconds, ever so gently releasing the pose the same way you got into the posture.
8. Walk the feet back in under the knees, unlace fingers and walk hands back. Come back to the crown of head and lower yourself down, one vertebrae at a time; the tailbone is the last part to connect back down to the earth.
9. Practice Knees to Chest or Resting Angel as you let everything relax down.

Modification

- Use blocks against the wall and/or on top of a non-slippery surface, or mat under hands and/or feet.
- Use blocks/prop under the elbows to elevate torso.
- Remain in Bridge until shoulders open and strength is gained.
- Use the seat of a chair, wrapping arms around the back of chair and lift your torso.
- Use an exercise ball, pillow, ottoman or similar prop to lay back on. Allow the heart to open and lift.
- Do not straighten the legs.
- Practice Fish.

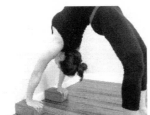
Blocks against the wall

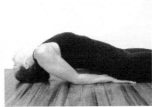
Fish

Wheel variation

Deepen

- Press into the earth, lifting entire front body toward the sky; engage entire legs and buttocks.
- Continue to use the breath to lift and expand energetically through the collarbone and the heart center.
- Extend one leg high, coming into Single Leg Bridge Pose and/or Shoulder Stand (Eka Pada Setu Bandha Sarnavgasana).

One Legged Bridge

Have you not known? Have you not heard? The Lord is the everlasting God, the Creator of the ends of the Earth. He does not faint or grow weary; His understanding is unsearchable. He gives power to the faint, and to him who has no might He increases strength. Even youths shall faint and be weary, and young men shall fall exhausted; but they who wait for the Lord shall renew their strength; they shall mount up with wings like eagles; they shall run and not be weary; they shall walk and not faint. Isaiah 40:28-31

BACK BENDING POSTURES

FISH (MATSYASANA)

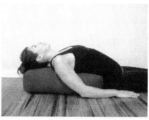

If any wound, offense, hurt, scar or walls have built up around your heart, allow this posture to open your heart once again. Be healed, renewed and restored. Exhale any residue of bitterness, resentment or wrongdoing. Inhale a new heart. Exhale the junk and inhale His Spirit to renew and mend.

Getting into the Posture

1. Starting in a supine position, come onto your elbows and tuck your fingertips under the buttocks or place the arms to the side as shown.
2. Rest the buttocks on the back of your hands as you press the elbows and forearms into the earth.
3. Legs are straight unless back issues are present.
4. You may also practice Fish in Lotus or Half Lotus leg position.
5. If legs are straight, actively engage the quadriceps up towards the sky.
6. Allow the scapulae to pull the elbows in towards the torso.
7. Gently lower the head opening up the throat and neck.
8. If the top of the head connects with the earth, there is not a lot of weight on the head itself.

Modification

- Bending legs will reduce tension on back.
- Keep chest closer to the earth.
- Use a block or folded blanket under the skull.
- Use blocks or a similar prop under the elbows.
- Place a folded blanket under the torso, stopping at your neck; let your head rest on the earth.
- Place a block or rolled-up blanket vertical with the spine, between the shoulder blades and allow your neck to hang off the edge as your collarbone lifts towards the sky.
- Gently hang head over the edge of your bed, maybe torso also.

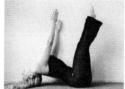

Rest on bolster lifting heart upward

Deepen

- Use Lotus or Half Lotus leg position. It is important to position legs first and then gently come down onto your elbows, then your back, to protect the spine from any injury.
- From fully reclined Fish, you can lift your torso towards the sky and grab for opposite elbows or extend both hands above your head.
- Practice Fish with arms and legs lifted (Matsyasana Variation).

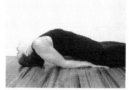

Tuck the fingertips under tailbone

Fish with arms & legs lifted

To further deepen practice...

UPWARD PLANK POSE (PURVOTTANASANA)

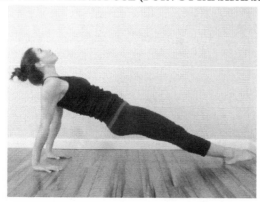

If you have no neck issues, head hangs backward as you lift the heart towards the sky. Inhale strength and calm. Exhale weakness. Inhale peace, exhale chaos. Like a fish, inhale life, freedom and joy.

He heals the brokenhearted and binds up their wounds. Psalm 147:3

Prayer:
Lord thank You that each day I am getting stronger and more flexible, not just physically, but in all ways. I am learning through stretching my faith that I can be pliable to everyday circumstances and that I can learn from all things, even from irritations. Things that use to annoy me have become lessons in patience. Thank You Father for stretching me and causing me to "grow up" in my spirit. I love You so much. May I be reminded through back bends to lift my heart and soul to You and sing to You a new song.
With all my heart, I will forever sing Your praises Lord.

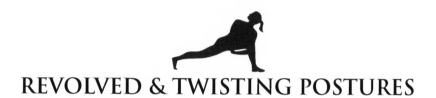

REVOLVED & TWISTING POSTURES

He said to me, "My grace is sufficient for you, for my power is made perfect in weakness."
Therefore I will boast all the more gladly of my weaknesses, so that the power of Christ may rest upon me.
2 Corinthians 12:9 English Standard Version

TWISTS

The greatest benefit of revolved postures is that they stimulate and cleanse every bodily system. This family of postures is the most renewing because it allows the body to be wrung out like a washcloth, massaging organs and stimulating systems. Twists can be as mild or as intense as you would like to practice. As the spine and surrounding muscles gain flexibility, your twists will become deeper, which in turn, cleanses and detoxifies even more.

The Word of God tells us that we must be renewed *daily*. Twisting postures cleanse us and can renew every fiber of our being. If you are like me, I have to be renewed several times a day!

Let's read this rich passage from the book of Romans.

Therefore I urge you, brethren, by the mercies of God, to present your bodies a living and holy sacrifice, acceptable to God, which is your spiritual service of worship. And do not be conformed to this world, but be transformed by the renewing of your mind, so that you may prove what the will of God is, that which is good and acceptable and perfect. For through the grace given to me I say to everyone among you not to think more highly of himself than he ought to think; but to think so as to have sound judgment, as God has allotted to each a measure of faith. Romans 12:1-3

There is so much in these few scriptures. It is vital that each day we renew our minds and cleanse our temples. Yesterday's thoughts, failures, and defeats *have to flee*. What brought us to where we are will not necessarily work in taking us to our destination. We must clear out the clutter and *create space for the new*. Twists physically, literally, spiritually and emotionally help detoxify every system so we can create space for new breath, the new "thing," new person, business, ministry or season. Going back to the cluttered garage scenario. Think of it like this: imagine a garage full of so much clutter that you cannot even park your car in it. Yet, you desire a new car. First, you cannot get the old car into a safe, warm, protected place. How do you expect a new car to come into your garage? You must de-clutter the garage and *make space* for the new things of God. You must take care of what you have, and clean out what you already have, before anything new can come in. It is the same concept with our physical, mental and spiritual bodies. It's time to put away the former things and press on to what lies ahead!

His master said to him, 'Well done, good and faithful servant. You were faithful with a few things, I will put you in charge of many things; enter into the joy of your master.' Matthew 25:21

We must first create space in every aspect of our lives and then God will be able to work within these new spaces. The larger the space the more room God has to do His work.

See, the former things have taken place, and new things I declare; before they spring into being I announce them to you. Isaiah 42:9

You can incorporate twists, or revolved poses, into almost every yoga posture, whether seated, standing, inverted, balancing, prone or supine. Revolved postures can be challenging. You will need patience in your journey with twists as they can be uncomfortable in the beginning. However, the more you practice these demanding poses the better you will become, so embrace where you are and enjoy the journey. You may need to press into the Lord and rely on His strength in some of these postures. Let Him show up when you need Him most. He tells us that His strength is perfected in our weakness, (2 Corinthians 13:9). So let go, and let God work in you.

Yoga twists increase the flexibility of your entire abdominal wall, including obliques and most back muscles. Inactivity can reduce the range of movement available to all your joints. Twists can assist in mobilizing the joints of your spine by rotating each vertebrae gently. Any revolved pose will squeeze the internal organs and encourage the flow of oxygenated blood, while eliminating toxins and metabolic waste products. The liver, kidneys, stomach, pancreas and spleen all benefit from twisting poses. Twisting poses can also help reduce abdominal bloating, digestive discomfort, menopause and menstrual symptoms. They may also be therapeutic for those that have an ulcer, hernia or are pregnant. What may be therapeutic for some may need to be avoided for others. As with any posture, twists can be as mild or as intense as you create them to be. Always ask a physician about any physical activity, especially if you have an ailment.

A twist will leave you feeling energized, focused, give clarity, relieve stress and deep tension. Remember to use props in the beginning. Sitting in a chair or using the back of a chair or a wall, can assist you in the beginning of your practice of revolved postures. As you breathe into the posture, your breath will help deepen your twist or explore any posture deeper.

EMBRACE WHERE YOU ARE AND ENJOY THE JOURNEY

Benefits of revolved postures include but are not limited to:
- Stimulates and massages the abdominal organs, including ovaries, prostate gland, bladder and kidneys.
- Improves and relieves digestion issues and tones the abdominal wall.
- Strengthens and stretches the back muscles, aligns and awakens the spine, improving posture.
- Stretches the hips, chest, shoulders, throat and spine, relieving tension in the back, neck and shoulders.
- Increases flexibility, lubricates ankle and knee joints while awakening the legs if extended.
- Stimulates heart and improves circulation.
- Therapeutic for mild sciatica, backache, arthritis, osteoporosis, menopause, menstrual discomfort and some infertility issues.
- Reduces stress and anxiety.
- Stimulates and energizes the circulatory, respiratory and nervous systems.
- Improves concentration, mental focus and relieves mild depression.
- Relieves mental and physical lethargy and exhaustion.
- Cleansing, calming, centering, balancing, brings a state of tranquility as well as can be invigorating.

Cautions include but are not limited to:
- Severe low back or shoulder injury.
- Ankle, hip or knee injury.
- Severe sciatica, degenerated or herniated disk(s).
- Third trimester pregnancy or severe diarrhea, ulcer, hernia, heartburn or indigestion practice modifications and/or avoid deep twists.

Revolved postures are a great way to start your day to remind yourself of this cleansing and renewal process. Remember, just like your walk with the Lord, these postures can start out uncomfortable and challenging. But enjoy the journey; breathe through these amazing and cleansing postures. Allow the Holy Spirit into your innermost parts to cleanse and heal you completely.

We are happy when we are weak but You are strong. We pray for this: that you will be made complete. 2 Corinthians 13:9

DIG IN THE WORD. YOUR SOUL WORK; 2 CORINTHIANS 12 AND 13 A MEDITATION FOR REVOLVED POSTURES

THE POSTURES

REVOLVED EASY POSE / GENTLE SPINAL TWIST (PARIVRTTA SUKHASANA)

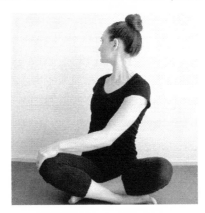

Preparatory Poses
- Child's Pose
- Simple Seated, Forward Folds or Staff Pose
- Garland
- Hero, Cow Face or Pigeon
- Side Stretches
- Bound Sage or Bound Angle Pose

Getting into Posture

1. From Simple Seated posture, gently turn the torso to one side, opposite hand anchors on the knee.
2. Lengthen through the torso; energetically the crown of head pulls upward and the tailbone is rooted to the earth.

Modification

- Place a rolled-up blanket under the tailbone to elevate spine and neutralize pelvis.
- Stay in Simple Seated without twisting.
- Sit on the edge of a chair, and use the back of the chair (or wall) to assist the core in rotating upper body.
- Use a block if needed under the hand that is behind the back.
- Another option for this posture is to drop your knees to one side, resting on the buttock and twist, keeping opposite hip and the knees on the earth (Sage Twist).

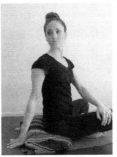
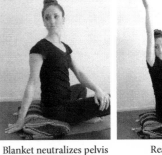

Blanket neutralizes pelvis   Reach arm

Breathe, twist and find your center in any variation. Anchor your thoughts on the Lord and breathe, going a bit deeper in the twist with each breath.

SAGE TWIST / SIMPLE SEATED TWIST (BHARADVAJASANA I)

All of the same great benefits, just a different variation. You may modify by placing a blanket underneath the hip that is on the earth. Take a bind or reach around to the opposite arm, you may also place one or both hands on a block.

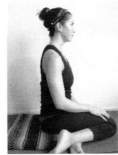
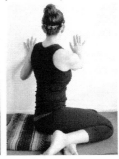
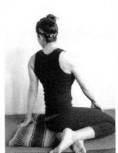

Blanket no twist   Use a wall   Blanket elevates tailbone

BOUND SAGE POSE / SEATED SPINAL TWIST I (MARICHYASANA C)

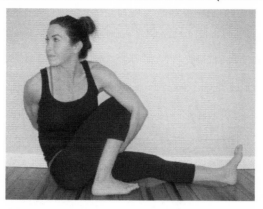

Getting into the Posture

1. From Staff Pose, bend one knee.
2. Clasp the opposite hand to knee or externally rotate and wrap opposite arm around the knee to bind and reach for the opposite hand (someday). Because your body is wedged against itself, you will most likely experience some restriction or a sense of confinement. Simply breathe through any discomfort, remembering never to force anything. We are always blessed when we press through the discomfort.

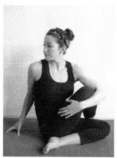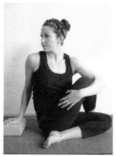

Practice with no bind   A block elevates floor

Stop trying to always be in control. Let it go with each exhale. As you inhale, focus on the opening, calming, balancing and rejuvenating effects of this pose. Inhale calm; exhale anxiety.

Yet another variation of this revolved posture is...

BOUND SAGE TWIST / SEATED SPINAL TWIST II (MARICHYASANA D)

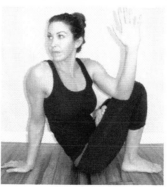

Getting into the Posture

1. From Sage Pose, come into Half Lotus with one leg, bend the other leg, bringing the opposite foot close to the hips.
2. Gently rotate the torso.
3. Lengthen your spine long and reach arm around for a bind, use a strap if necessary or simply place elbow on the exterior of knee. Leg can also be on earth as opposed to Half Lotus position.

Modification

- Don't bend the knee.
- Use a strap around the foot that is in hip crease or for a bind with the hands.
- You may also place a blanket under the tailbone to elevate and neutralize the pelvis and spine more.

Practice another variation…

MARICHI'S POSE II / SEATED SPINAL TWIST (MARICHYASANA II)

Getting into the Posture

1. From Staff Pose, bend one leg so the sole of the foot is planted on the earth, or Half Lotus into the hip crease.
2. On the same side as the bent leg, that arm extends up to lengthen the spine; torso then forward folds while the extended arms reaches to the inside of the bent inner thigh.
3. From the forward fold, the extended arm externally rotates around the outside edge of the bent thigh.
4. The opposite arm externally rotates, one day clasping the other hand or fingers for a bind.

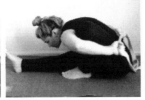

Modification
- Stay upright.
- Sit on a folded blanket or block.
- Use a strap and/or blocks.
- Practice Simple Seated Twist.

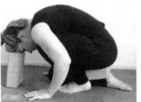 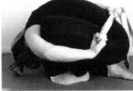 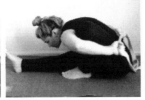 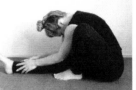 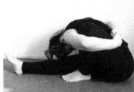

| Sit on block and rest forehead | Use a strap to assist the bind | Straighten leg with strap | Lessen the fold no bind | Straighten leg with bind |

Deepen
- Add a twist.
- Open the arms and shoulders.
- Reach further; try grasping opposite elbows.
- Hold for one minute, and switch sides.

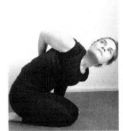 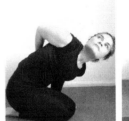

Twist and open   Open arms

HALF BOUND LOTUS TWIST (BHARADVAJASANA II)

Getting into the Posture

1. Place one foot in the opposite hip's crease.
2. You may place hands on floor or blocks as well as take a bind. You may also use a strap until shoulders open enough to grasp for the foot.

Breath is relaxed as you breathe into the shoulders and hips; let the upper back tension melt away as you enjoy the calming and centering effects of this posture. Always center your heart and mind on Christ. Allow Him to always work on your behalf. Inhale the fact that all you need to "do" is just believe. Trust. Rest.

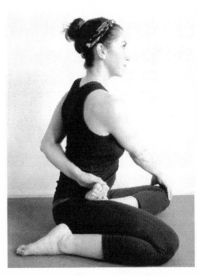

You may also extend the foundational leg and come into...

SPINAL TWIST IN HALF LOTUS (ARDHA PADMA MATSYENDRASANA)

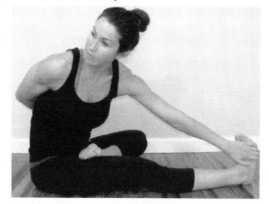

Choosing the same variation, modification or to deepen this posture as mentioned in Half Bound Lotus Twist.

Breath is relaxed and you enjoy the opening and invigorating effects of this posture.

Deepen
- Continue to use each exhalation to deepen the twist. Hollow out the belly more and more.
- Deepen the bind by further reaching and/or folding.
- Deepen the twist with every exhalation.
- Place a block at the foot of extended leg and reach to the edge of block.

Be careful to never force rotation. The lumbar spine can only twist five degrees around the vertical axis. Using a body part or limb instead of the core center to help you in rotation can cause serious injury.

Practice another variation...

SEATED HALF SPINAL TWIST / HALF LORD OF THE FISH (ARDHA MATSYENDRASANA)

Getting into the Posture
1. Tuck one foot under one leg as you bring one knee upright towards heart center.
2. Whichever side the upright knee is on, this hand is placed palm down behind you as you gently twist the torso.
3. Allow the back hand to act as a "kickstand" to keep spine lengthened.
4. The opposite elbow rests on the interior of the upright knee.

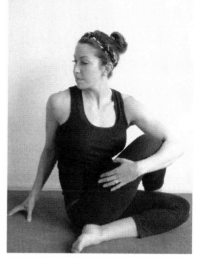

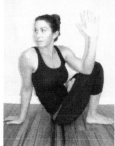
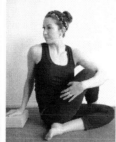

Modification
- Place a rolled-up blanket under the tailbone to neutralize pelvis and spine.
- Do not twist or lessen the twist.
- Place hand that is behind body on a block.
- Sit on the seat of a chair and use the back of the chair to help support you. The abdominal is doing the work; don't allow the hand to fully turn your torso to injure your lower back.
- Sit on a blanket; place hands on a wall for a mild twist.

Lessen the twist   Place block under palm

Deepen
- Continue to use each exhalation to deepen the twist. Hollow out the belly more and more.
- Be careful to never force rotation. Use only the core muscles to rotate the upper body.
- Practice a bind with arm reaching behind to rest in the crease of hip, further opening the shoulders, chest and neck. Gently release the pose by twisting in the opposite direction.

RECLINING SPINAL TWIST (JATHARA PARIVARTANASANA)

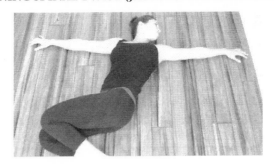

Getting into the Posture

1. Begin by lying on your back, bending your knees into a 90-degree position.
2. Airplane out your arms to the sides, palms facing down.
3. Using your oblique and core muscles, gently lower both knees to the ground.
4. Attempt to keep both shoulders planted on the earth.
Create space on the opposite side of the knees by drawing the shoulder and ear away from each other.
5. Turn your gaze away from the knees, looking beyond the fingertips.
6. Focus on drawing the navel in towards the spine and the mobility of the spine as you twist. For a more restorative posture, relax the abdominal muscles.

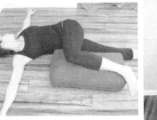
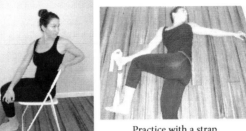

Bolster keeps hips in alignment

Mild twist in a chair

Practice with a strap

Modification

- Gaze stays forward, as opposed to looking at the opposite side of knees.
- Place a rolled-up blanket under the tailbone.
- Place a blanket between the ground and bottom thigh.
- Place a block, pillow or bolster between the thighs.

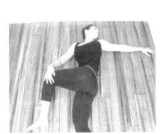
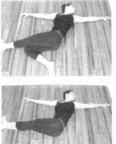
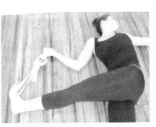

Assist the knee for a deeper twist

Extend one or both legs

Use strap with extended leg

Deepen

- Continue to use each exhalation to deepen the twist. Hollow out the belly more and more. Do not force rotation.
- Gaze towards the opposite hands, both palms down.
- Lengthen the top leg reaching for the ankle or use a strap and reach for the strap.
- You may also bring the arm (the same arm of the extended leg) over the head and reach for the strap or foot, breathing into the rib cage, pulling the navel towards the spine.
- Both legs extend out, energetically engaged throughout the entire body, press the heels out and away from midline.

REVOLVED SEATED FORWARD FOLD (PARIVRTTA PASCHIMOTTANASANA)

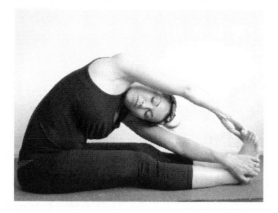

Getting into the Posture

1. From Staff Pose, hinge at the hips into a forward fold.
2. Grab for opposite foot, opposite hand.
3. Turn your torso inward and outward toward the opposite foot.
4. Continue to open the rib cage and try to keep the legs connected with the earth as much as possible.
5. Continue to use your exhalations to open up the throat, neck, shoulder, chest and heart center.
6. Pull the navel into the spine and massage your internal organs with every breath.

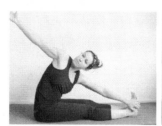
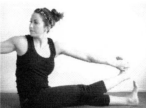
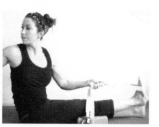

Lessen the twist   Reach for the exterior of foot and   Practice with a block under leg and
lessen the twist   a strap

Modification

- Place a rolled-up blanket under the tailbone.
- Place a blanket under the knees, or simply bend both knees.
- Use a strap around the soles of the feet and only forward fold, do not twist. Lead with your heart in the fold.
- Reach behind you without folding, wrists of both hands in alignment as you hold one foot and extend the other hand behind you, reaching energetically with each finger.
- Keep one leg bent; reach only one arm or both arms as you turn your torso upward.

Deepen

- Continue to use each exhalation to deepen the twist and open up the side body.
- Be careful to never force rotation.
- Reaching opposite hand and foot, lift the foot and leg as you twist.
- Breath is steady. Let the rib cage expand as you inhale. As you exhale, let your tension release.
- Allow your thoughts to calm, center and focus.

Close your eyes. Meditate on the fact that you are exactly where you are supposed to be. It may be uncomfortable, but that's okay. Breathe. You are almost there. Feel yourself arrive in this posture. Inhale flexibility and strength. Exhale anything else. Inhale Him. Exhale you.

SEATED GATE (VIRA PARIGHASANA)

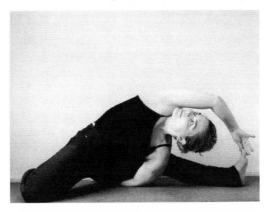

Getting into the Posture

1. From Staff Pose, bend one knee back, allowing the heel to rest near hip, top of the foot is on floor.
2. On an inhalation lengthen the torso, on an exhalation use the core muscles to bend sideways toward the extended leg as you reach the arm around the back of the head to connect to the toes or foot.
3. The other hand may tuck under the thigh as shown, rest on the thigh or simply rest on the earth.

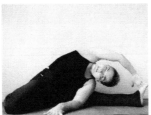
Extend arm

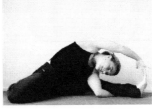
Head to knee with arm under extended leg

Modification

- Do not extend leg out long, keep knee bent or place block/blanket underneath.
- Place a rolled-up blanket or block under the knee(s).
- Reach arm upward instead of over the head to the foot.
- Use a strap around the extended leg's foot.
- Use a block against the wall to press the extended foot into.
- Sit on a chair, extend one leg out and add a side bend to the opposite side.

Deepen

- Continue to use each exhalation to deepen the twist and the fold, open up the entire body and focus breath on the side body.
- Breath is steady. Let the rib cage expand as you inhale.

As you exhale, any worry or fears subside. Close your eyes. Center your thoughts. Inhale stamina and perseverance; exhale weariness and insecurities. With each breath, allow your lungs and heart to open up to the Lord.

REVOLVED STANDING FORWARD FOLD / WIDE A-FRAME FORWARD FOLD
(PARIVRTTA PRASARITA PADOTTANASANA)

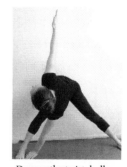

Getting into the Posture

1. From Mountain Pose, airplane arms out to the side as you step out wide.
2. Hinge from the hips, coming into a forward fold.
3. Reach one hand to the exterior of the opposite foot. You may also place hand in front center or on a block.
4. Extend other arm upward, energetically reaching for the sky.
5. Hollow out the belly.

   Think of wringing yourself out like a washcloth. That is what you are doing as you twist; you are massaging and cleansing your internal organs.

Modification

- Lessen the forward fold and/or practice without twisting.
- Place blocks under each hand, keeping spine elevated and heart lifted.
- Keep a micro bend in the knees.
- Elevate the heels with a rolled-up blanket or similar prop.
- Rest forearms on a chair, with or without a twist.

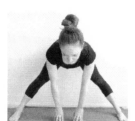
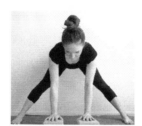
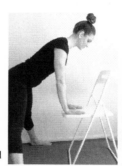
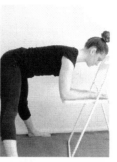

Half way fold with no twist   Place blocks to elevate the floor and lift the spine   Use the seat of a chair   Forearm on seat

Deepen

- Continue to use each exhalation to deepen the twist and the fold; open up the entire body and focus breath on the side body. Both wrists are in alignment.
- Use only the core muscles to rotate the upper body.
- Press the tailbone back, creating a flat "tabletop" with the spine.
- Reach the fingers that are extended towards the sky energetically.
- Breath is long. Take time to absorb the many benefits of this full body posture.

Deepen the twist, hollow out the belly

   As you exhale, deepen the posture and breathe out things or relationships that no longer serve you. Create space for new things, new relationships and a new perspective. As you inhale, bring in those new things. Inhale the good; exhale the not-so-good. Make sure to repeat just as long on the other side. Inhale the new season and pathway, exhale the old journey. Surrender your past to the Lord; allow your future to be in the hands of the One who creates all things, including your future!

Prayer:
Heavenly Father, thank You that I am fearfully and wonderfully made!

REVOLVED & TWISTING POSTURES

REVOLVED SIDE ANGLE (PARIVRTTA PARSVAKONASANA)

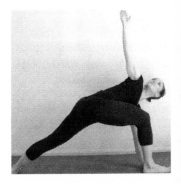

Getting into the Posture
1. From Side Angle, replace the inner hand that is on the earth with the extended hand.
2. Using the core, rotate the torso and reach upward and backward. Pull the navel in towards the spine.
4. Gaze can be up at the extended hand or down at the ground.
5. Try to keep all four corners of both feet rooted to the earth and continue to press through the knife edge of the back foot engaging the entire leg. It's okay to be elevated on the toes of the back foot.

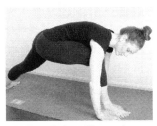

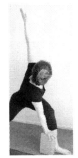

Modification
- Place foundational hand on block or similar prop.
- Place support under the back heel to elevate it and assist with support and balance.
- May use a block against the wall or the wall itself to brace the back foot for support.
- Use a chair for support, practice a mild twist or no twist at all.

Face the leg with no twist

Elevate hand with a block

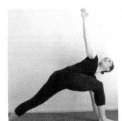

Deepen
- Continue to use each exhalation to deepen the twist.
- Torso is lifted and buoyant, not resting on the front leg.
- Press all four corners of both feet into the earth; energetically lift the hamstring of the back leg towards the sky.
- Remember, never force rotation. The lumbar spine can only twist five degrees around the vertical axis. Using a body part or limb instead of the core center to help you in rotation or any revolved posture can cause serious injury. Use only the core muscles primarily to rotate the upper body.

Energetically reach, stacking the wrists

Breathe through the uncomfortable feelings. Focus your thoughts on your strongest self. Embrace and honor the journey of the path that you are on. It is not always easy or comfortable, but it is always worth it. Inhale truth. Exhale the things that are not truth.

You can also come into…

BOUND SIDE ANGLE POSE (BADDHA PARSVAKONASANA)

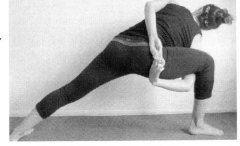

Getting into the Posture
1. Untwist from Revolved Side Angle, come into Side Angle, and deepen the lunge slightly.
2. With the arm placement in front of the lunging thigh, internally rotate and reach back through your thighs with the opposite arm externally rotating and reaching behind the tailbone one day connecting for a bind, focusing on "rolling open" the top shoulder. As you breathe in this expression, focus on lifting the heart towards the sky and expanding the lungs and chest.

I will lift up my eyes to the mountains; from where shall my help come?
My help comes from the Lord, who made heaven and earth. Psalm 121:1-2

REVOLVED & TWISTING POSTURES
MOUNTAIN TWIST (PARIVRTTA TADASANA)

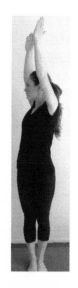

Getting into the Posture
1. From Mountain Pose, inhale arms up (or you may keep them on hips), biceps by ears.
2. Turn your torso to one side, keeping the legs strong, active and engaged.
3. Turn towards the other side and hold as long as you did on the other side; thighs always stay facing forward.
4. You may also flow from side to side with the breath.

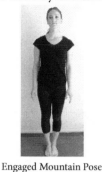
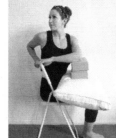

Modification
- Keep arms by side; focus on engaging the legs.
- Close your eyes.
- Stay in Mountain, feeling the stabilizing and calming effects of Mountain.
- Place feet hip-width apart and engage the entire lower body without twisting.
- Sit at the edge of chair and use the back for a mild twist.

Engaged Mountain Pose   Chair twist

Deepen
- Inhale to lengthen spine in center Mountain, raising biceps near ears, exhale twist to one side, flowing with each breath.
- Continue to use each exhalation to deepen the twist.
- Close your eyes as you move or as you stay on one side.
- Incorporate side bends or back bends, see variations shown.

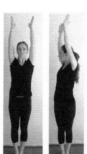
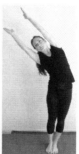
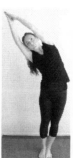
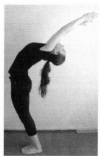

REVOLVED CHAIR (PARIVRTTA UTKATASANA)

Getting into the Posture
1. From Mountain Pose, feet together or hip-width, deeply bend both knees to come into Chair; keep shoulder blades back and downward. Look down and make sure you can see your toes. If you cannot, sit back further.
2. Hollow out the belly, using only the core muscles twist the torso to one side, the elbows only act as an "anchor" lightly on the exterior of the knee.
3. Hands can be at heart center, arms raised so that the biceps are near the ears or open the arms wide to the side.
4. You may find more stability with your feet together. If so, engage the ankles, knees and thighs together.

Modification
- Lessen the twist and/or depth of bent legs.
- Place foundational hand on block or higher elevation (Chair, bench, etc.).
- Place support under the back heel to elevate it and assist with support and balance.
- Stay centered in chair; do not twist.
- Sit on the edge of a chair and use the back of a chair to mildly twist.

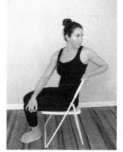
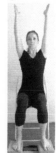
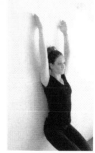

Chair seated twist   Extend arms in chair   Use a wall

Deepen
- Continue to use each exhalation to deepen the twist.
- Torso is lifted and buoyant, not resting on the front leg.
- Spine lengthens with each inhale; do not curve or cave into the thighs.
- Outstretch your arms long, opening your heart and shoulders to the sky.
- Press all four corners of both feet into the earth; knees and inner thighs connect.
- Practice Side Crow arm balance from Revolved Chair.

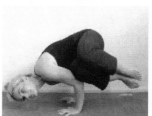
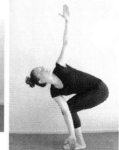

From Revolved Chair come into
Side Crow

Outstretch the arms wide

REVOLVED TRIANGLE / PYRAMID (PARIVRTTA TRIKONASANA)

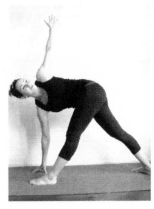

Getting into the Posture

1. From Triangle, bring the top arm to the inside of the front foot or the exterior of the foot, for more of a challenge, try to get fingers and toes flush.
2. Gently rotate the torso inward.
3. Extend the hand that was to the interior of the foot back and upward. Energetically engage the arms and keep alignment from wrist to wrist. Use a block under the hand on the ground to elevate spine if needed.
4. Remain buoyant and lifted in the torso, one day lifting the foundational hand off the earth.
5. Energetically lift the knees and thighs; draw the inner thighs together.
6. Draw the navel in towards the spine.

Modification

- Lessen the twist.
- A narrower stance can help stabilize and support balance more.
- Place foundational hand on block(s) or higher elevation such as a chair.
- Place support under the back heel to elevate it and assist with support and balance.
- Practice Triangle without twisting.
- Rest on the edge of a chair and use the back of a chair for a mild twist.
- Do not twist.

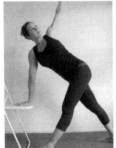
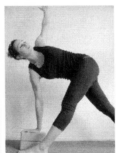
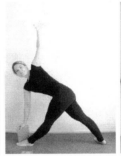
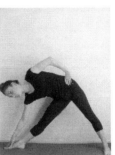

| Use the seat of a chair to elevate spine | Use one or more blocks | Use blocks at various heights | Arm on hip, no twist |

Deepen

- Continue to use each exhalation to deepen the twist.
- Torso is lifted and buoyant, not resting on the front leg.
- Spine lengthens with each inhale; do not curve or cave into the thighs.
- Outstretch your arms long, opening your heart and shoulders to the sky.
- Press all four corners of both feet into the earth, (especially) root the back heel down.
- Use the core center to lift hand off the earth.

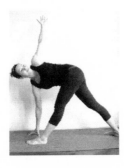

REVOLVED & TWISTING POSTURES

To further deepen the expression and challenge your balance you may come into...

REVOLVED HALF MOON POSE (PARIVRTTA ARDHA CHANDRASANA)

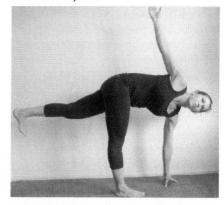

Getting into the Posture

1. From Revolved Triangle, lift the back leg. Use a block under hand if needed.
2. Roll hips open, back leg someday parallel to the earth.
Healthy necks look up towards the outstretched hand; otherwise, gaze stays down or straight ahead. Breathe.
3. Perhaps lift the bottom hand off the ground someday.

This posture can be challenging in the beginning. I recommend using a wall, chair, and/or a block for either the back foot or the front hand to help as you improve your balance. As you strengthen your muscles and flexors, not only will your balance improve, but also this posture improves and develops concentration, willpower, focus, stamina and determination. Balancing postures can be the most difficult of asanas but they are extremely beneficial and important as we age. Any balancing posture will improve stability, which can prevent falls, injuries or bone breakage if we do fall.

Never practice moving in and out of externally and internally rotated femur poses (Revolved Half Moon into Half Moon). It places too much pressure on the head of the femur of foundational leg, and may cause serious injury or breakage of the bone.

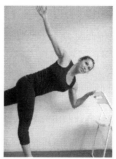 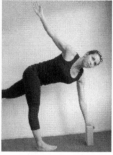

Use a chair for stability Use blocks at various heights

Embrace the challenges of this pose and life. Find something still to gaze upon. Calm your thoughts and steady your heart. Inhale grace and exhale grace. Allow His grace to be extended to others around you. You cannot give what you do not contain.

REVOLVED CRESCENT / REVOLVED HIGH LUNGE (PARIVRTTA ANJANEYASANA)

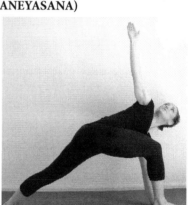

Getting into the Posture

1. From Crescent Lunge, bring the back hand to the interior of the front foot or the exterior for more of a challenge. You may also use a block or the seat of a chair for support.
2. Turn the torso upward as you extend the opposite arm behind you.
3. Keep both feet firmly rooted to the ground.
4. Gaze is down, forward or up towards the fingertips, wherever the neck is comfortable.

Modification

- Lessen the twist and/or depth of bent legs.
- Place foundational hand on a block or the seat of a chair.
- Place support under the back heel to elevate it and assist with support and balance.
- Stay centered in Low Lunge with knee on earth or Crescent (High Lunge).

Deepen

- Continue to use each exhalation to deepen the twist.
- Energetically lift the back hamstring towards the sky.
- Torso is lifted and buoyant, not resting on the front leg.
- Spine lengthens with each inhale; do not curve or cave into the thighs.
- Outstretch your arms long, opening your heart and shoulders to the sky.
- Press all four corners of both feet into the earth.
- Lift hand off ground.

Each inhale brings in strength. Each exhale eliminates self-doubt. Inhale God-confidence!

Finally, be strong in the Lord and in the strength of His might. Put on the full armor of God, so that you will be able to stand firm against the schemes of the devil. Ephesians 6:10-11

NOOSE (PASASANA)

Getting into the Posture

1. From Mountain Pose, take a deep bend in the knees, squatting low as the tailbone and heels connect. May use a wall for assistance.
2. Gently swing the knees to one side and turn your torso slightly to the opposite side.
3. Externally rotate both arms to meet near the small of your back for a bind.
4. Engage the arms into the torso.
5. Press all four corners of both feet into the ground. May also use a blanket under heels if you find them lifting.
6. Gaze is where the neck is comfortable.

Modification

- Place the front hand on the ground for more stability.
- Place a rolled-up blanket under the heels to assist with balancing.
- Only wrap one arm around one leg, don't come into the final binding stage.
- Use a strap to assist with the bind, until one day your shoulders open up enough to clasp for the hand, wrist, or forearm of the opposite arm.
- Sit on a chair, thighs parallel to earth; you may need blocks under both feet, then place right hand to the outside of left thigh or on the back of the chair or wall.
- Breathe and work up to turning and folding the right side torso onto the thigh.
- Make sure to perform the same amount of time on the left side.

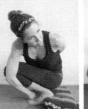
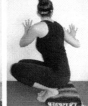
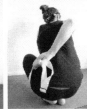

Blanket elevates the heels   Wall for stability   Strap assists the bind

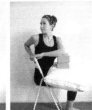

Use a chair and a wall   Chair with mild twist   Chair gentle twist

Deepen

- Continue to use each exhalation to deepen the twist. Never force rotation.
- Continue to lift the heart towards the sky; lengthen the spine, twist and lift.

Release fear of the unknown. Get comfortable with being uncomfortable. Inhale calm; exhale distractions. Continue to steady your heart and thoughts on Him and ease into this amazing posture that has innumerable benefits. Continue to reach new depths in this pose. Inhale diligence, exhale failure.

If we say that we have no sin, we are deceiving ourselves and the truth is not in us. If we confess our sins, He is faithful and righteous to forgive us our sins and to cleanse us from all unrighteousness.
If we say that we have not sinned, we make Him a liar and His word is not in us. 1 John 1:8-10

With every twist, inhale the Lord and all His benefits deep into your soul. Allow twists to cleanse your systems so you will be made whole. As you explore the depths of these postures, allow your heart to be completely surrendered and able to take in all that He will speak to you as you relax into a posture. Remember, you will create great space for new things. Allow Him to speak those *new* things to you.

That the God of our Lord Jesus Christ, the Father of glory, may give to you a spirit of wisdom and of revelation in the knowledge of Him. I pray that the eyes of your heart may be enlightened, so that you will know what is the hope of His calling, what are the riches of the glory of His inheritance in the saints, and what is the surpassing greatness of His power toward us who believe. These are in accordance with the working of the strength of His might. Ephesians 1:17-19

Prayer:
Dear Heavenly Father, thank You for every trial and tribulation that has sharpened me, matured me, and caused my life to glorify You. Just as some of these challenging postures are not always easy or comfortable, so as it is with my walk with You. Through it all Lord, this is what I know for sure, that you are a faithful God. You created the Universe, yet I can climb into your lap and call you Daddy! Thank you for cleansing me. Renewing me. Pruning those things and people that no longer belong in my life. It's not easy. It doesn't feel good Lord, but I know that you have done this and will continue to shake loose all the things that no longer belong in my life. For this, I simply say thank You. Thank You for always having my best interest at heart. Your plans are for my good. Never to harm me, always to prosper me. How can I say thank You? I just want my life to thank You. To glorify You with every breath I take. I love you, Father. In Your Son's precious name, I pray all these things. Amen and Amen!

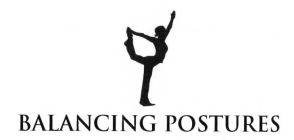

BALANCING POSTURES

*To focus our minds on the human nature leads to death,
but to focus our minds on the Spirit leads to life and peace.* Romans 8:6

BALANCING POSTURES

Oh, the subject of balance! It seems so elusive, doesn't it? Do you long for more balance in your days? Are the pressures of life exhausting you and sucking your time down the drain? Do you have balance in any area of your life? How does one do it all and still find peace, rest, space, and time for loved ones *and* time with the Lord? We have our home life, kids, and chores. Then we have to make a living. We have our work life with all its demands and pressures. We must balance work life and home life. It's a challenge to keep work at work and not bring it home. Another challenge is if you work from home, or are a full time stay at home mom or dad. What about children's many extracurricular activities? What about important relationships? Church? Serving? Missions? The list goes on. We are exhausted from the list and anxious just thinking about it. There are only seven days in a week and we are supposed to rest on one of these days. We're already off to an unfair start, working six days and resting one. If we don't feel exhausted at the end of the day, then we feel like we're failing or missing the mark. The truth is we need rest and we need to create a more balanced and joyful life.

In this chapter, you'll do more than learn about balance and the importance of obtaining balance in your life. You may actually begin to *experience* a balanced lifestyle. Learning about balancing postures can help us remain focused, centered and find strength in not just a posture, but for daily life. When we learn how to breathe, relax, focus, concentrate and find mental clarity in a posture, we can take these elements far beyond a yoga mat.

What does the Word of God say about the subject of balance? I think it is important to look at the beginning. In Genesis, we read that God created and formed the Universe and all that is within it and even what is outside of it. He did all of this in six days. But, on the seventh day, He rested. Keep in mind that God did not rest because He was exhausted; God never tires. God was setting an example for us to follow. He took one day to look at what He had done, to rest and to say, "It is good." If rest is important to God, why would we think that rest is not important to us?

With all the innovations and gadgets to make our lives more simple and fast, why don't we have enough time? We should have time to have dinner with those who are closest to us. We should have more time to invest in important relationships, family, community, serving others and much more. What keeps us so busy? As mentioned, "B.U.S.Y is defined as *Buried Under satan's Yoke.*" This has never been truer than today. I look at my grandparents' generation, they had time to cook, eat together, play together, vacation together and so much more. They did it all without the help of electronic gadgets to "simplify" their lives or make things "easier" and "faster." I believe we need to get back to basics if we are going to find true balance in our lives. It is important to find rest from all of our activities, but also ensure those activities are things that we value, are productive and align with God's will for our lives.

The following activity can help you get on the road to balance.
• List your current activities and interruptions. Don't leave anything out.
• Think about the future, your family and other relationships.
• Think about your core value system and the eternal value of each activity in your life.
• Then, using a scale of 1 to 4 – with 1 being the most important use of your time, and 4 being the least important use of your time – place a number next to each activity (1's will be non-negotiable; work, school, etc.).
• Next, cut out all "Number 4" activities from your life. Presto! Gone!

It can be that simple, really! This will create margin and space for activities that are more meaningful for rest and the balance you need. Of course, you can revisit those "Number 4" activities, but maybe lay them aside for a season. You may find that you don't miss those things at all, or more important, they were not productive toward your higher calling.

An activity that can create more balance in your life is to serve others. We are not busier than Jesus himself was, are we? Throughout the Bible, we see how Jesus, no matter what, always had (or made) time for others. How often do we read in scripture, "...*While he was on his way, He stopped...?*" Numerous examples in the Bible show how Jesus allowed time for interruptions. We need to create enough space and margin in our days to be interrupted. With zero margin or time for interruptions we become frazzled, burned out, stressed, angry, and downright no good to ourselves or anyone around us. Besides, interruptions often turn into divine appointments. If we are so busy rushing around, interruptions are annoyances, and we have no patience or room for grace toward others. This causes us to be unlike Christ more than anything else. Allow interruptions in your life. You'll see, the Lord will indeed bless you as you bless others with your time.

If you ever feel overwhelmed, just ask your Father what you might need to cut out of your life. Ask Him. He will speak to your heart, but first you have to get still, be quiet and simply ask. Unless you are quiet, you will not be able to hear Him when He does speak. In everything under the sun there is a season (Ecclesiastes 3:1-8). Trust that His will is going to happen in your life. You can't do a thing to speed it up or diminish it.

Being confident of this very thing, that He which hath begun a good work in you will
perform [it] until the day of Jesus Christ. Philippians 1:6

Be well balanced (temperate, sober of mind), be vigilant and cautious at all times; for that enemy of yours, the devil, roams around like a lion roaring [in fierce hunger], seeking someone to seize upon and devour. I Peter 5:8 Amplified Version

BALANCING POSTURES

It is easy to become unbalanced. Our bank accounts can suffer if we are not financially balanced or keeping track in this area. Over-shopping or obsessive thriftiness can cause stress and frustration. Our bodies may be exhausted because we are not balanced in taking care of ourselves. We can err on the side of too much exercise or no exercise; neither is healthy. We may spend too much time with our children and not enough time with our spouse. Being unbalanced in this area can create pressure and frustration in these relationships. Too much time working and not enough time resting will affect every area of your life.

For most of us, our days are spent being extremely unbalanced and off kilter. This is exactly how the enemy would want us to remain: *busy.* When we get unbalanced, the enemy sneaks in an open door where we are not paying attention. We can be so focused on certain things that we lose sight of other things, which is why it is important to remain balanced.

Remaining balanced requires maintenance and rechecking your activities and priorities often. Balance means keeping things in a *harmonious arrangement,* or as Webster's defines it, "a state of just proportion." Seek to be balanced and *maintain* your balance in every area of your life. Just like a vehicle, checkup and maintenance is required.

BALANCING POSTURES

Meanwhile, the moment we get tired in the waiting, God's Spirit is right alongside helping us along. Romans 8:26

Balancing postures will improve mental focus, clarity, concentration, memory, and coordination, while developing strength and stability. They can also reduce tension, anxiety, depression, and fatigue. Each balancing posture strengthens different joints and muscles in the body. Standing balancing poses build strength, while lubricating the foot, knee, and hip joints. Arm balancing postures strengthen the entire arm, including hands, wrists, and shoulders, while also lubricating and increasing mobility in all these joints. All balancing postures strengthen the core center.

Balancing postures focus on the micro muscles, tendons, ligaments, and our joints, which are important to improve and maintain as we age to prevent injuries. Practicing balancing postures not only lessen the chances of injury, but if we do fall or experience an accident of sorts, there is less injury or breakage because these postures actually strengthen our joints and bones. Because balancing postures require a great deal of strength, it is a good idea to use props and tools in the beginning to assist with postures. A wall, chair, or block(s) will assist you into a safe, effective, and well-aligned pose.

This particular posture family requires a great deal of concentration; it is the perfect opportunity to turn your heart and mind towards the Lord. Fix your gaze on Him; remain steadfast, sturdy, and strengthened! In these postures, you will deepen your understanding of what is required to have balance, not just in postures, but also in your everyday life. Balancing postures require great strength, but also tender softness. Just like these two opposites, our lives and walk with the Lord are full of juxtapositions. The elements in this chapter will help you reclaim your balance. Have patience with balancing poses. They can be challenging, and will only come with time and practice. Also, allow yourself grace as you learn balancing elements for your life. Change can often be uncomfortable and can get us agitated, but breathe through the change. Allow yourself grace as you grow in becoming more like Christ by creating balance in all areas of your life. Transformation is a process and it never happens overnight.

Use these postures to inhale stability and balance as you exhale imbalances. Each inhalation continues to reach to new heights and possibilities; each exhale releases fears and self-doubt. Allow His grace to wash over you so that you can extend grace to others. Create margin for divine interruptions in your life.

Benefits of balancing postures include, but are not limited to:
- Strengthens the back muscles, thighs, calves, ankles, feet and arms.
- Relieves flat feet.
- Stretches inner thighs, groins, shoulders, chest and hips.
- Lubricates and increases mobility in foot, knee and hip joints.
- Stretches and tones the back of legs and gluteal muscles.
- Improves alignment of the spine improving posture.
- Improves circulation, digestion, constipation, gastritis, menstrual and menopause symptoms.
- Therapeutic for mild sciatica, osteoporosis and tension backaches.
- Improves balance, strength, coordination, mental clarity and concentration.
- Relieves fatigue, anxiety and depression.
- Strengthening, rejuvenating and calming.

Cautions include but are not limited to those with:
- High or low blood pressure (practice modifications).
- Headache, insomnia, vertigo, sinusitis, glaucoma, arthritis or fibromyalgia.

DIG INTO THE WORD. YOUR SOUL WORK; ROMANS 8, THE MESSAGE
A MEDITATION FOR BALANCING POSTURES

THE POSTURES

TREE POSE (VRKSASANA)

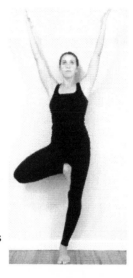

Preparatory Poses
- Forward Folds, Mountain, Chair
- Bound Angle and other hip openers
- Warrior I, II, III or Reverse Warrior
- Triangle or Side Angle
- Reclining or Seated Pigeon
- Cow Face, Stretching Tiger

Getting into the Posture
1. From Mountain Pose, shift your weight onto one foot, and root down into all four corners of that foot.
2. Bring the sole of the opposite foot into the ankle, above the kneecap, or to the interior of the standing leg.
3. Engage the foundational leg as you lift the torso tall, keeping the shoulder blades back and down.
4. Slightly tuck the sacrum under and straighten out the waistline.
5. Place palms at heart center, "cactus arms," or extend your arms (branches) towards the sky, keeping shoulders back and down, away from the ears.

Modification
- Keep hands by side or at heart center, palm pressed together.
- Stand against a wall.
- Keep lifted leg against opposite ankle or above the knee (Never on the knee joint).
- Only lift the foot off the floor slightly or place toes on a block, until balance improves.
- Place both or one hand on a wall, perhaps work up to not using the wall.
- Use the back of a chair to support yourself.

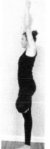 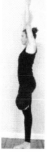 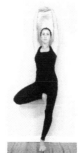

Hands to heart center   Toes to ankle   Use a prop such as a chair

Deepen
- Raise arms above head.
- Interlace fingers and press palms up.
- Close your eyes.
- Look up and/or add a back bend.
- Include lateral flexion by side bending.

Counter poses
- Mountain
- Back bends
- Forward Fold, Half-Way Fold
- Shoulder Stand, Inversions
- Arm Balances
- Child's Pose
- Resting Angel

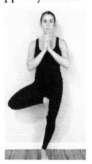 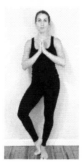 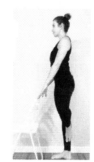 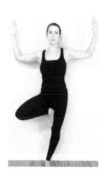

Arm variations   Add lateral flexion

STANDING HEAD TO KNEE (DANDAYAMANA JANU SIRSASANA)

The purest definition of influence is a solid and strong character. Would you be kind to yourself, and accept that you are solid and strong in the Lord? Remind yourself that because you possess these characteristics, they brew in your soul, there is no space for failure and defeat. You have influence. You are strong! God created you to be more than a conqueror. This means beyond victorious!

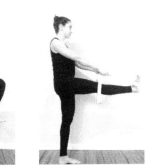

Getting into the Posture
1. From Mountain Pose, bring one leg into the chest and interlace all ten fingers around the bottom of the foot.
2. Engage the foundational leg as you pull the navel in towards the spine; gently extend the leg in front of you.
3. Allow the spine to round over the leg as you keep the leg as straight as possible.
4. Bring the forehead to the knee; elbows hug the exterior of the leg for full expression.

Modification
- Do not forward fold, just clasp around the foot, or use a strap.
- Instead of extending leg out, gently lift the toes to the ground or a block until balance improves (see Tree Modifications).
- Stand against a wall.
- Practice Tree.
- Start with the wall, and begin to move away from using the wall.
- Set extended leg on a chair or bench.
- Practice while seated in a chair.

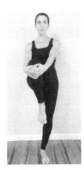
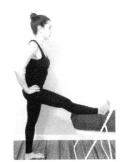
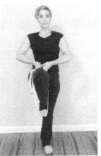
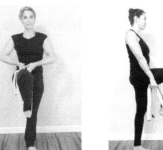
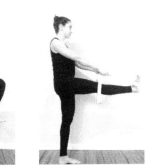

Stay upright   Use a prop such as a chair   Practice with strap and variations

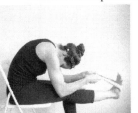

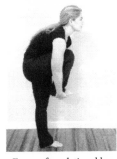

Practice seated with a strap

Deepen
- Leading with the heart, forehead is secondary, hinge forward, elbows melt down to the sides of knee.
- Hold for a minute before switching sides.

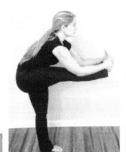
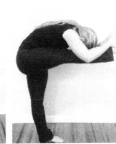

Engage foundational leg   Extend leg, use core   Forehead to knee

EXTENDED HAND TO TOE POSE (UTTHITA HASTA PADANGUSTHASANA)

Inhale evenness and harmony as you exhale instability in this posture. Feel the sensations of being rooted and grounded. Embrace being uncomfortable and settle your heart and mind from any anxious thoughts. Steady your thoughts on Christ.

Getting into the Posture

1. From Mountain Pose, bring one leg into the torso while engaging the standing leg.
2. Clasp the exterior of the foot with the same side hand and extend forward.
3. Take a couple of breaths to find your stability then bring the leg out to the side. Simultaneously, the opposite arms extends out, palm down, gaze beyond the fingertips for full expression. Keep the foundational leg forward and strong.

Modification

- Keep hands by side or at heart center, palm pressed together.
- Stand against a wall.
- Keep knee bent; arm may extend upward.
- Practice Tree Pose.
- Only lift the foot off the floor, or toes on block, until you improve your balance.
- Set extended leg on a chair, bench, or wall; hands center or on hips.
- Use a strap around foot of extended leg.
- Keep the extended leg out front.
- Bring leg out to the side but keep gaze forward.
- May place hand on the hip as well.

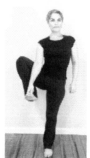 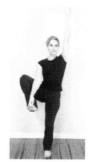

Do not extend leg   Stay center raise one arm

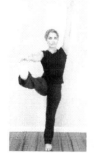 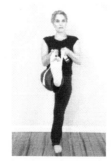 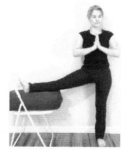 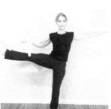 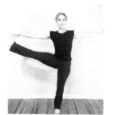

Extend to front only   Front and strap   Use props such as chair and wall   Use strap, look forward   Look forward

Deepen

- Look the opposite direction of extended leg; engage the foundational leg.
- Hold for a minute before switching sides.
- Bring extended leg further upward.
- Flow from Tree into Extended Hand to Toe.

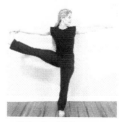

Bring leg higher, gaze opposite direction

BALANCING POSTURES

HALF MOON POSE (ARDHA CHANDRASANA)

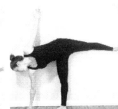

Inhale centered-ness. Really feel what it feels like to be centered and stable in your mind, body and spirit. Inhale that from the fingertips to the toes. Say to yourself, "I am stable. I am confident. I am strong in the Lord."

Getting into the Posture
1. From Triangle Pose, slightly bend the front leg as you lift your back leg, energetically pressing through the heel.
2. The lower hand is placed in alignment with the exterior of foundational foot (Pinky toe and thumb should align).
3. Allow your hips to gently "roll" open as you straighten the front leg without hyper-extending the knee and pull the navel in towards the spine.
4. Extend the upper arm high, energetically "sparking" the fingertips, gaze beyond the hand.
5. Work up to holding Half Moon for 30 seconds or longer.
6. Release by coming back into Triangle, Mountain or Standing Forward Fold, practice on the other side.

Modification
- Stand against a wall.
- Foundational hand is on a block or use the wall. Set the block up to the tallest height and eventually as you improve your balance, the block will disappear.
- Place the extended leg's foot on the wall.
- Use the wall for support with either the hand, foot or back.
- Gaze is down or forward as opposed to upward.

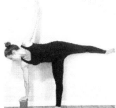
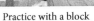
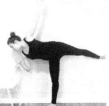

Practice with a block   Use a chair and/or stand against the wall   Place palm on earth, gaze down, forward or upward

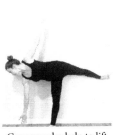

Core muscles help to lift hand off earth

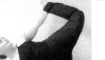

Half Moon variation

Deepen
- Lift the hand off the floor or block, engaging the entire body and core to do so.
- Extend the top hand out energetically, wrist to wrist is in perfect alignment.
- Close your eyes.
- Bend top leg and grab for the foot for a variation.
- Place the hand with the thumb in alignment with the standing leg's pinky toe.

REVOLVED HALF MOON (PARIVRTTA ARDHA CHANDRASANA)

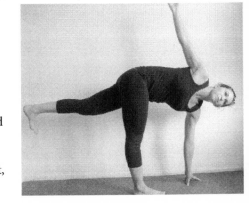

Caution: Practice Half Moon and Revolved Half Moon separately, as opposed to flowing into Revolved Half Moon from Half Moon. Internally rotated femur postures should not move into externally rotated femur postures as the weight of the body is too much pressure for the femur.

Getting into the Posture
1. From Warrior III, hips are squared to the earth in this posture; place the opposite hand of the foundational leg to the interior (or exterior for more of a challenge) of the foot.
2. Float the opposite arm towards the sky as you rotate your torso, keeping leg lifted.
3. Continue to press through the heels. Elongate the spine and breathe, opening the chest, lungs and heart.

Inhalations bring in resilience, power and energy. Exhalations expel lack, fear, weakness and cowardice. You can do all things through Christ who strengthens you!

I delight in weaknesses, in insults, in hardships, in persecutions, in difficulties.
For when I am weak, then I am strong. 2 Corinthians 12:10

BALANCING POSTURES
EAGLE POSE (GARUDASANA)

Each inhalation will bring in poise and grace, as your exhalations will cleanse you of instability and insecurity. Find your strongest self in this fierce posture. Focus on the Lord. Embrace the centering and groundedness as you root down in Christ. Forge ahead into freedom. What does freedom look like in your life? Allow your mind to be free. Allow your physical body to free. Receive your healing in this new found freedom.

Getting into the Posture

1. From Mountain Pose, inhale as the arms extend upward; press the palms together.
2. Swing your right hand under your left arm. Wrap the elbows, forearms, wrists and palms and/or fingers.
3. Exhale into a deep squat as if you are coming into chair pose; come onto the right toes as you shift your weight into the left foot, simultaneously lowering the arms so hands are in front of face.
4. Wrap the right thigh on top of the left thigh, pointing your toes to one day wrap behind the left calf.
5. Drop the shoulders back and down, create space between the ears and shoulders.
6. Make sure your alignment is straightened, everything is facing forward, straighten out the waistline.
7. Hold for up to 30 seconds. Release back into Mountain, give yourself a gentle back bend and practice on the other side.

Modification

- Place toes on a block, as opposed to wrapping them behind foundational leg.
- Sit or kneel and only practice Eagle Arms to open the shoulders.
- Lessen the bend in the knees.
- Stand with tailbone against a wall.
- Keep arms down, at heart center or on hips.
- Practice upper body and lower body separately before combining.
- Wrap your hands behind your shoulders, giving yourself a hug instead of coming into Eagle Arms.
- Simply cross the legs instead of wrapping them.

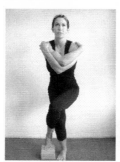 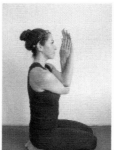

Place block under foot,   Sit with Eagle Arms
only wrap arms

Deepen

- Thighs are parallel to the earth.
- Forward fold as you pull your shoulder blades back, down, and apart as your elbows stretch forward, coming into "Sleeping Eagle." The knees and elbows connect. Hollow out the belly and gaze at elbows.
- Flow with your breath in and out of Eagle and Warrior III; keep core engaged and proper alignment.

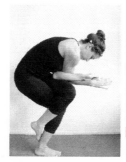 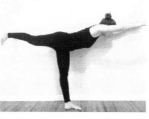

Flow from Sleeping Eagle into Warrior III

WARRIOR III (VIRABHADRASANA III)

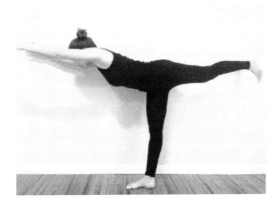

Inhale tolerance and persistence, as you exhale indifference and timidity. As you come into your deepest expression of this strong, fierce pose, remind yourself that you are a survivor full of courage and perseverance. You have come this far and you won't stop now. Remain focused on the Lord, sturdy and steadfast.

Getting into the Posture
1. From Mountain Pose, inhale arms above the head.
2. Step one foot out, slightly bending the knee for protection, as you simultaneously lift the back leg.
3. Squaring the hips towards the ground, hinge at the hips and bring the torso halfway down.
4. Attempt to create a "T" shape. Gaze is a couple feet in front of you as you energetically pull the biceps close to the ears and bring them backward.
5. Shoulder blades are back and down.
6. Hold for up to 30 seconds, gently bend the front knee stepping back into Mountain and repeat on the other side.

Modification
- Lessen the hinge.
- Use blocks underneath both hands.
- A wall or chair supports either your front hand(s) or back foot.
- Airplane the arms out to sides.

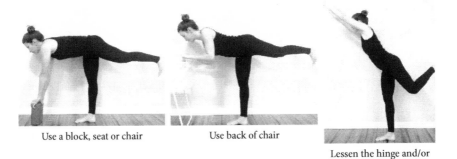

Use a block, seat or chair   Use back of chair

Lessen the hinge and/or use a wall

Deepen
- Energetically "hug" every muscle to every bone as you come into your deepest expression.
- Reaching towards the front as your back leg is energetically pulling away (Reach in opposite directions).
- Without touching the floor, come into Eagle Pose, add a flow with these two postures.
- Flow in and out through Warrior I to Warrior III.
- Flow in and out through Warrior III and Eagle.
- Come into Standing Splits.

STANDING SPLITS (URDHVA PRASARITA EKA PADASANA)

Inhalations bring in energy and life. Your exhalations send out tiredness and things that no longer serve your physical, mental, emotional and spiritual well-being. Inhale zeal and vitality, and exhale ineffectiveness and inability. Repeat to yourself, "I am able. I can do all things through Christ. I am okay being moved, changed and reaching a new standpoint. I am gaining a new outlook and perspective on everything around me." Take in new energy in your deepest expression of this wonderful posture. Allow the Lord to stretch your faith!

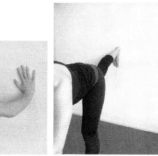

Getting into the Posture
1. From Mountain Pose, inhale to upward salute as you exhale come into a Standing Forward Fold. You may also come from Warrior III or Single Leg Swan. Use your exhale to bring your torso closer to the legs.
2. Wrap one arm or elbow behind the same calf.
3. Extend the opposite leg up as much as possible. Keep the hips somewhat squared and engage the entire body.
4. Allow the head to hang heavy with no tension in the neck.

Modification
- Lessen the hinge.
- Bend the supporting leg.
- Use blocks under both hands or keep both hands on the floor.
- A wall or chair supports either your front hand(s) or back foot.
- Airplane the arms out to sides.
- Keep back leg on ground.
- Practice Warrior III, may also use blocks with Warrior III.

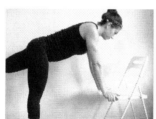
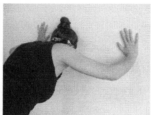

Practice with a chair   Practice with a wall

Deepen
- Energetically "hug" every muscle to every bone as you come into your deepest expression.
- Let your exhalations help you hinge forward as your heart comes closer to the front leg; let the head "hang heavy".
- Wrap one or both arms around the supporting leg; forearm(s) embraces the lower leg, perhaps elbow hiding behind the calf.
- Torso connects with thigh.

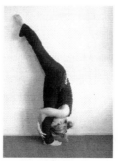

Arms wrap

BALANCING POSTURES
SINGLE LEG SWAN BALANCE (EKA PADA HAMSA PARSVOTTANASANA)

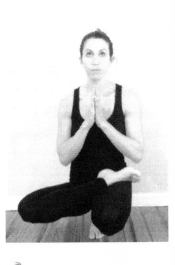

Getting into the Posture
1. From Warrior III (or Standing Splits), bring the palms to prayer position into heart center, or reverse prayer behind you to open the shoulders. Keep your gaze out in front of you and focus on something still.
2. Continue to press through the back leg, flexing the back foot, keep a straight line of engagement.
3. Keep hips squared to the earth, lift through your heart center upward. Use blocks or bring reverse prayer to front prayer.

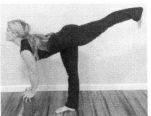
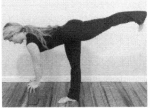

This posture will continue to challenge your balance. Inhalations bring in grace, exhalations carry out harshness and imbalances. Lift your heart toward the Lord.

Add a block   Head down

TIP TOE POSE (EKA PADANGUSTHASANA)

Inhale tolerance and gentleness in this posture. Exhale brokenness and fractures. Your inhalations will create space for healing as your exhalations take you further into the unknown and force you to trust. As you exhale, let the walls you've built simply melt. Inhale being yielded, surrendered and vulnerable once again. Trust again here in this pose. Trust God.

Getting into the Posture
1. From Mountain Pose, bring one foot into the crease of the opposite hip joint.
2. Bring palms together at heart center.
3. Begin to sit back as if you were going to sit into a chair. When your torso begins to come forward, you may release your fingertips to the ground for support.
4. In a deep squat, bring your tailbone to the heels while coming to the toes of the foundational foot.
5. Come to your fingertips, then place one hand, or both hands for full expression, to the heart center as you balance on your toes.
6. Practice holding the posture up to 30 seconds, then come into an arm balance or release the posture back into Mountain Pose and practice on the other side.

Modification
- Keep foundational heel elevated with support of prop under heel.
- Keep both hands on earth, the tallest height of block, or only one hand to heart center.
- Stay in Half Lotus Forward Fold or halfway point.
- After tailbone drops towards heels, keep both hands on ground, blocks, chair or wall.

Place hands on chair   One hands stays on earth

Deepen
- Bring both hands to heart center.
- Close your eyes.
- Hinge forward and come into an arm balance, Flying Pigeon (Eka Pada Galavasana), perhaps extending the back leg out, engaging the entire core and backside body, especially the glutes and hamstrings.

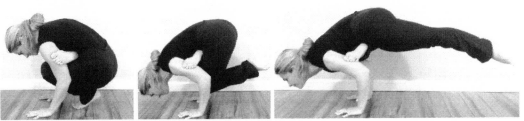

Deep forward fold   Arm Balance   Flying Pigeon
Arm Balance prep

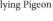

BALANCING POSTURES
STANDING HALF BOW / DANCER (UTTHITA ARDHA DHANURASANA)

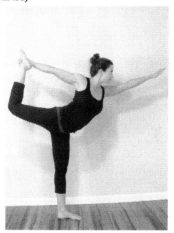

Inhale determination, exhalation laziness. Focus on releasing idleness. Continue to bring in assurance with each inhale, reminding yourself that you are strong, able, creative and willing. Inhale this truth as you lift your heart and gaze up and forward. As you exhale, you are cleansing your mind of myths and lies about yourself. Breathe in the truths of what God says about you!

Getting into the Posture

1. From Mountain Pose, bend one leg so that the heel and buttock are close or connected. This same hand clasps for the ankle as you bring the knees back together and in alignment.
2. Inhale and bring the opposite arm above the head, palm facing outward.
3. Reach for the interior of the bent leg's foot, ankle, or shin. You may also use a strap.
4. Energetically kick into the hand, drawing the thigh and heel away from the buttock. Kicking is the "engine" in the posture.
5. When you can no longer "kick away," hinge at the hips as the torso comes forward. Simultaneously, the extended arm lowers down in a straight line pointing forward with the palm down.
6. The front palm comes in alignment with the nose and mouth.

Work up to holding posture 30 seconds or longer. Repeat on other side.

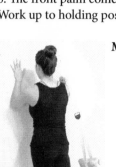

Modification
- Lessen the back bend.
- Use a wall or chair for support.
- Use a strap around the foot or ankle.

Use a wall and/or strap

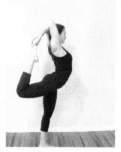

Deepen
- Continue to lift the heart towards the sky.
- Deepen the hinge from the hips.
- Both hands connect with back foot as you engage the foundational leg.
- Straighten out the back leg, perhaps both legs vertical someday.
- Practice Lord of the Dance or both legs extended.

Both hands clasp foot

LORD OF THE DANCE (NATARAJASANA)

In Lord of the Dance, straighten both legs as much as possible.

Dancing is poetry in motion. As you achieve your deepest expression of Dancer, this pose will loosen your inhibitions, rules and expectancies. Instead, free the artist, creator and performer in you that may have been dormant. Reach further with each inhalation, reach for the moon!

Let your exhalations release any rigidity. Trust the Lord to see you through all transformations!

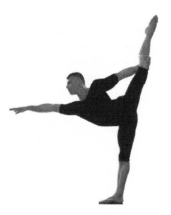

We find ourselves standing where we always hoped we might stand—out in the wide open spaces of God's grace and glory, standing tall and shouting our praise. Romans 5:2 The Message

BALANCING POSTURES
ONE LEGGED GARLAND POSE (EKA PADA MALASANA)

Find your center in this pose. Feel the impressions of being focused. The feeling of achievement and success. Inhale victory and triumph. Inhale being proud but exhale pride and ego.

Getting into the Posture

1. From Garland Pose, lengthening through the spine and sitting tall, extend one arm up and behind you as you lift your gaze towards the outstretched hand.
2. The opposite hand extends and is energetic toward the ground, broaden your chest and open the shoulders and heart center.
3. Place the extended upper arm behind the back (use a strap if needed) and let the lower arm reach for the other hand; come into a bind by interlacing all ten fingers or grabbing the strap. This brings your gaze forward and down.
4. Bring the leg that is not in the bind to center and under the body. Shift your weight onto this foot.
5. Inhale as you lift your torso, simultaneously engaging the arms around the bound leg, and lift everything upward. Press through the heel of foundational leg and broaden your chest while lifting your heart up.
6. Hold up to 30 seconds, gently release exactly as you came into the posture and repeat on the other side.

Modification
- Practice Garland or Noose.
- Use blocks under both hands or keep both hands on the floor.
- Practice Garland with a mild twist and/or bind with a strap if needed.
- Use a chair and strap.
- Practice Warrior III or Bird of Paradise.

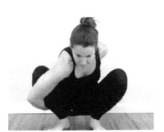
Garland with bind

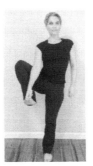
Stand with grabbing toe

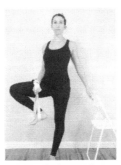
Stand with chair and strap

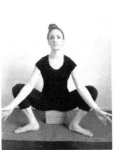
Use blocks

Deepen
- Energetically "hug" every muscle to every bone as you come into your deepest expression.
- Let your exhalations help you hinge forward and your heart come closer to the front leg.
- Torso connects with thigh, or front knee connects with armpit.
- Incorporate a twist into posture for Revolved One Legged Garland.

To further deepen practice...

REVOLVED ONE LEGGED GARLAND (PARIVRTTA EKA PADA MALASANA)

Hug the knee into the chest as you twist deeply from the core center (If you lift your left knee, then twist to the left).

BALANCING POSTURES
BOAT POSE (PARIPURNA NAVASANA)

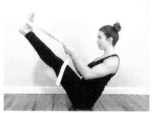

Inhale composure, exhale imbalance and impurities in this posture. Find steadiness and equilibrium in the full expression of Boat. Steady your thoughts on Him. Focus on not letting the things around you into your boat. If they do splash in, vow to keep your peace and calm.

Think on all those things which are pure, lovely, and of good report. Philippians 4:8

Getting into the Posture

1. Sitting on the ground with knees bent, remove any excess flesh so you are directly on the sitting bones and tailbone.
2. Bring your feet off the floor and extend your arms toward the feet.
3. Pull the navel into the spine; lift the chest tall, keeping a straight spine in this posture.
4. Extend the legs out long.

Modification

- Bend knees.
- Wrap hands behind thighs for additional support.
- Use a strap around the soles of the feet.
- Do a classic sit-up.
- Practice One Legged Boat (Ardha Eka Pada Navasana). Only one leg extends out, while the other is on the ground. Knee is bent or extended.

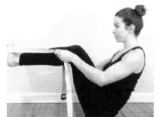
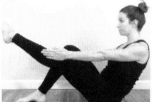
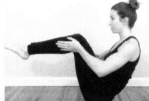
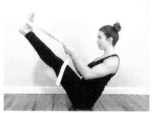

Bend knees with or without strap   One Legged Boat   Bent knees   Straighten legs with strap

Deepen

- Lift through the heart center, chin lifted, space in between throat, outstretched hands.
- Clasp hands at back of head and extend legs out or just extend legs wide.
- Flow from Boat to Canoe or hold up to a minute.
- Practice Double Toe Hold (Ubhaya Padangusthasana).
- Practice Canoe by lowering the limbs closer to the earth.
- Practice Upward Facing Forward Fold Balance (Urdhva Mukha Paschimattanasana), where torso and forehead connect.
- Practice Open-Leg Seated Balance Pose (Urdhva Upavistha Konasana).

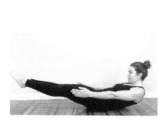
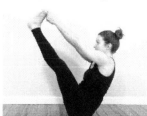
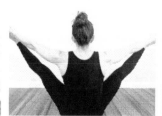
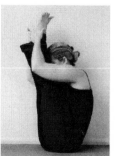

Canoe   Double Toe Hold   Open-leg Seated Balance Pose

Upward Facing Balance

Inhale distractions into your life as a *good* thing. Take time for divine interruptions along the way and be elevated because of them. Inhale and release the to-do lists and agendas; exhale your need to be in control at all times. Inhale flexibility and pliability, exhale rigidity. Allow the Lord to transform you here, remembering that transformation is a process.

Further progressing, practice...

FETUS POSE (GARBHASANA)

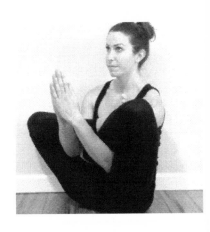

Getting into the Posture
1. From Open-Leg Seated Balance Pose, stay upright as you come into Lotus or Half Lotus Legs. You may also cross the legs to your comfort level.
2. Bring arms through, elbows to the inner thighs and bring your hands together (or try other hand variations).

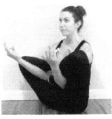

Deepen
- Close your eyes.
- Bring your knees to touch the torso.
- Practice on the palms for an arm balance; torso upright, gaze forward.

Hand variation

Building yourselves up on your most holy faith, praying in the Holy Spirit. Jude 1:20

Also try...

BALANCING BOUND ANGLE (DANDAYAMNA BADDHA KONASANA)

In the deepest expression of this posture, realize that you are free from any interruptions or obstruction. No obstructions stand between you and your destiny! Keep diligently seeking out this posture. Continue to challenge yourself in this pose; surrender to fear and frustrations. Exhale frustration and inhale calm.

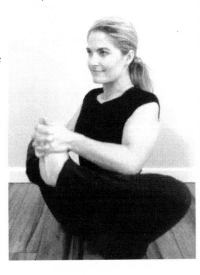

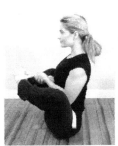 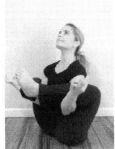

Getting into the Posture
1. From a seated position, bring the soles of your feet together and interlace the fingers on the outer edge of the feet.
2. Keep your torso tall as you bring the feet to heart or chin level.
3. Press the legs into the arms or simply "hug" everything inward energetically. Keep the chest open and the heart lifted by rolling the shoulder blades back and down.

Use a strap   Hands under legs

Enlarge the place of your tent, stretch your tent curtains wide, do not hold back; lengthen your cords, strengthen your stakes. Isaiah 54:2

Prayer:
Dear Heavenly Father, today I simply praise You for giving me wisdom to create space for You, my family, and other valuable things in my life. Help me never lose sight of how important it is to create time and space for these things. I want every relationship in my life to honor You. I am never more fulfilled that when I am a servant. Show me where I can serve You and Your people. I know that when I fill my day with serving, the funniest thing happens; I have all kinds of time on my hands! Help me to enjoy my life and my many blessings. Guide me to be a blessing to others and to stop taking everything so seriously. You are light, joy and peace. Thank You for a balanced life in You.
Amen and Amen!

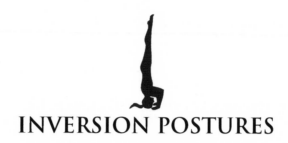

INVERSION POSTURES

Keep me as the apple of your eye, hide me in the shadow of your wings. Psalm 17:8

INVERSION POSTURES

Though you have made me see troubles, many and bitter,
you will restore my life again; from the depths of the earth you will again bring me up. Psalm 71:20

Sometimes we get used to looking at life through our individual filters and lose sight of the proper perspective, and more important, *God's perspective* and what He might be trying to get to us through a circumstance or person. Read the following passage of scripture, written by Paul to the "holy ones in Christ Jesus;" that is you and me!

But whatever were gains to me I now consider loss for the sake of Christ. What is more, I consider everything a loss because of the surpassing worth of knowing Christ Jesus my Lord, for whose sake I have lost all things. I consider them garbage, that I may gain Christ and be found in Him, not having a righteousness of my own that comes from the law, but that which is through faith in Christ— the righteousness that comes from God on the basis of faith. I want to know Christ—yes, to know the power of His resurrection and participation in His sufferings, becoming like Him in His death, and so, somehow, attaining to the resurrection from the dead. Not that I have already obtained all this, or have already arrived at my goal, but I press on to take hold of that for which Christ Jesus took hold of me. Brothers and sisters, I do not consider myself yet to have taken hold of it. But one thing I do: forgetting what is behind and straining toward what is ahead, I press on toward the goal to win the prize for which God has called me heavenward in Christ Jesus. All of us, then, who are mature should take such a view of things. And if on some point you think differently, that too God will make clear to you. Only let us live up to what we have already attained.

Join together in following my example, brothers and sisters, and just as you have us as a model, keep your eyes on those who live as we do. For, as I have often told you before and now tell you again even with tears, many live as enemies of the cross of Christ. Their destiny is destruction, their god is their stomach, and their glory is in their shame. Their mind is set on earthly things. But our citizenship is in heaven. And we eagerly await a Savior from there, the Lord Jesus Christ, who, by the power that enables Him to bring everything under His control, will transform our lowly bodies so that they will be like His glorious body. Philippians 3:7-21

In this chapter we will study inversion postures. I love inversions because they remind me to gain a *new* perspective. The whole world, literally and figuratively, turns upside down in these physical (and sometimes demanding) postures.

Have you ever had your world turned upside down? Sometimes, all you have to do is simply gain a new perspective on an old situation. Inversions are stimulating and energizing. They *restore* and *revive* all of your bodily systems. To revive is to *reawaken*. Do you need to be revived or awakened? Fan the flame, even if it is small, awaken a new perspective, and revive your mind, body, spirit, and soul.

In the above passage, Paul reminds us that the things we once thought so important can be lost. But it is okay, because for everything I lose, I gain with, and in, Christ. Paul calls the old things "garbage." Is your old way of looking at things or perhaps those important earthly possessions *garbage*? He is saying that as we mature and grow *in* Christ, so does our perspective. Or at least the hope is that we mature in Christ and grow up spiritually. Not that we obtain perfection or holier-than-thou status, but we can rest in the promise that we can move forward and begin to write a *brand-new* script. You can press on and push forward to a higher calling. His power will enable you, *if* you receive the calling.

But our citizenship is in heaven. And we eagerly await a Savior from there, the Lord Jesus Christ,
who, by the power that enables Him to bring everything under His control,
will transform our lowly bodies so that they will be like His glorious body. Philippians 3:20-21

My prayer for you during this time is that you dust yourself off and begin again. Sometimes we have to stir ourselves up. This takes energy and courage. You need these two things to press on toward the prize and high calling. Inverted postures also require energy and courage. Do not be intimidated by inversions. You always need courage and energy to try something new, but inversions will assist in giving you more of these two things. We are never more blessed than when we get out of our comfort zones and attempt something new.

God's ways and thoughts are much higher than ours are. We cannot comprehend His vast love, mercy, kindness and grace. Usually for God to get us where we need to be, it is a difficult and lonely process. He strips away the things that no longer belong in us or around us. He shakes loose those people, places and circumstances that we no longer need as He molds, conforms and transforms us from the inside out. This transition, or development of character, can be extremely painful. But just like inversions, we gain a new outlook and perspective in life through these uncomfortable, agitating and pruning seasons. Things that never made sense to us come into clarity.

Jesus, the ultimate example, prayed for His enemies and treated them with kindness. Jesus never spoke negatively to those who wished Him harm. Even though He committed no sin, He was attacked, sworn at, spit on and nailed to a cross. Still, He spoke kindly and prayed for those who oppressed Him. In the natural realm, this does not make sense. In reality, there are times when we would like to "lay hands" on our enemies, and not in the prayerful way, if you know what I mean. But God prays for and loves His enemies.

INVERSION POSTURES

His grace never runs out. Every day His mercies are fresh in your life. Grace piled upon grace; this is His amazing love for you.

Whether you are developing yoga postures or deepening your walk with Christ, growth and maturity come easier with practice. Perhaps now you can get one step closer to being Christ-like. Think of an enemy, or someone who has done wrong toward you. Now, lift that person up in prayer. Say, "Father, I pray that you would bless _____ today (I know, ouch on the first time around!). I ask that you would cover them, protect them, and send your Holy Spirit to speak to them that they would have ears and a heart to hear from you." Simple enough, right? Praying for your enemies requires a *new perspective*. But...you survived! It may be difficult for you at first, but I promise it will become easier. You will be blessed beyond your wildest imagination by imitating God and doing things opposite of your flesh. You will be more blessed when you do the right thing, even though you do not *feel* like doing it. Now, preparing a dinner and sitting at the table with thine enemies may come later, or maybe just in Heaven, but congratulations! You are growing and becoming more like Christ!

This leads us to inversions. Perspective, patience, difficulty, challenges, pain, resistance, revival, renewal, perspective and becoming more like Him are all processes and a transformative season. You can expect all of these things – plus peace, joy, and content- ment – during this time. I dare you to let go of whatever has kept you from moving forward and reaching your destiny. The time is now. The place is here, and *you*, my friend, are *the one*!

INVERTED POSTURES

Inversions typically have the heart, and often the feet, elevated higher than the head. Many inverted postures stimulate every bodily system, which revitalizes, restores and rejuvenates. If you suffer from depression, anxiety, fatigue, stress, asthma or other respiratory and circulatory deficiencies (depending on the severity), then you will want to incorporate inversions into your everyday life. It could be something as simple as placing your legs up a wall or on the back of your headboard after a long day. These postures can be as mild or as intense as you choose. Because inversions are so energizing, practicing deep inversions before trying to sleep is not recommended. Mild inversions are fine, as they can also calm and restore. Explore and enjoy the countless benefits of inversions.

The cardiovascular benefits of inversion postures improve circulation through fresh delivery of blood to the heart and other organs. Being inverted also increases blood flow to your head, relieving the heart of some of its duties and can in turn, lower blood pressure and an overactive heart rate. Being inverted creates great circulation around the eyes and cheeks, which can greatly improve the texture, tone and elasticity of your complexion. Some people notice less wrinkles and improved facial tone after practicing inversions each day.

Your endocrine system is responsible for hormone delivery. Inversions, especially shoulder stands, are recommended for peri-menopausal and menopausal women due to the belief that the postures stimulate the thyroid and parathyroid glands. Stimulating these glands also results in an increased metabolism. If you have other hormonal issues, just as with any asana practice, ask your doctor. A shoulder stand may be beneficial for one person and may be the opposite for another practitioner. Know your limitations. It is good to challenge yourself and try new things but never force a posture; always listen to your body. It will tell you things, do not ignore those promptings.

Nervous system benefits of inversion postures include the stimulation of cerebrospinal fluid, or CSF, the fluid of the central nervous system that flows from the brain into the spinal cord. In a headstand specifically, the top of the skull experiences pressure that promotes elasticity in the cranial bones. This increases the production of CSF to the ventricles of the brain and stimulates thought process, creativity and more.

Let inversions revive your soul! Dedicate these poses to Him and invite His Spirit to do a cleansing work in your body, mind and heart. It is a good idea to absorb the labor of these postures by ending in a relaxed or restorative posture such as Child's Pose, Restorative Fish or Resting Angel. As you relax and surrender, allow Him to speak to you during the silence. You will be awakened, alert and attentive to His voice in the stillness of this new space that you create to hear from Him.

Benefits of inversions include but are not limited to:
- Improves and relieves digestion issues.
- Tones the entire core.
- Stimulates the thyroid and parathyroid glands; increases metabolism and stimulates the nervous, digestive, lymphatic, circulatory and respiratory systems.
- Strengthens and stretches the back muscles, aligning spine and improving posture.
- Relieves backaches and tension, specifically upper back, neck and shoulders.
- Opens the shoulders and chest.
- Awakens the entire lower body, specifically the hamstrings, calves, glute muscles and feet.
- Stimulates the heart and improves circulation.
- Allows the heart to rest from stressful duties.
- Can be therapeutic, or you may need to avoid if high or low blood pressure or diabetes is present.
- Therapeutic for menopause discomfort, infertility, insomnia and sinusitis.
- Can prevent headaches and sinusitis.
- Can be therapeutic for asthma, flat feet and sciatica depending on the severity.
- Reduces stress and anxiety.
- Increases energy and stamina.
- Improves concentration, mental focus and relieves depression.
- Relieves mental and physical exhaustion.
- Invigorating, strengthening and healing.

Cautions include, but are not limited to:
- Back, neck, elbow or shoulder injury.
- Severe sciatica, herniated disk or carpal tunnel syndrome.
- Third trimester of pregnancy, diarrhea, hernia, ulcer, glaucoma, vertigo or severe asthma.
- High or low blood pressure, heart issues or diabetes.
- If you are menstruating, menopausal or have fertility issues, practice modifications or avoid deep inversions.

Prayer:
Thank you Father, for tuning my ear to hear You even though the place or space is new and uncomfortable. I am grateful that You strengthen me as you prune things from my life. Thank You for allowing this space for new things, new perspectives, and new ways to look at things, especially when You literally get me upside down. No matter where I am or what I'm doing, may I represent You well. Amen!

DIG INTO THE WORD. YOUR SOUL WORK;
PSALM 71 THE MESSAGE
A MEDITATION FOR INVERSIONS

THE POSTURES

Do you have eyes but fail to see, and ears but fail to hear? And don't you remember? Mark 8:18

DOWNWARD FACING DOG (ADHO MUKHA SVANASANA)

Preparatory Poses
- Child's Pose
- Forward Folds
- Son Salutations
- Legs up the Wall
- Shoulder Stand
- Planks or Dolphin Pose

Getting Into the Posture
1. From a Standing Forward Fold, walk your hands and feet outward; bend your knees as much as you need to in the beginning.
2. Become an inverted "V" shape, with hands and feet about hip-width apart.
3. Shoulder blades roll back and down your back as the tailbone lifts upward. Pull the navel towards the spine while energetically gripping the earth with the fingers outward. Imagine you are unscrewing the lid of a jar. Right fingers energetically "grip" outward to the right, and left fingers "grip" outwardly to the left.

Modification
- Place a block against the wall and press hands or feet into blocks.
- Rest forehead against or on a bolster or block.
- Use blocks under hands.
- Keep knees bent.
- Practice Dolphin (Ardha Pincha Mayurasana). To *deepen Dolphin*, add a strengthening flow by crunching the knee to nose or elbow; or flow from Dolphin to Sphinx.

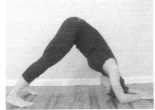
Dolphin

Sphinx

Deepen

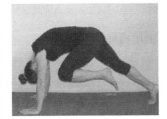

Three Legged Dog to a knee crunch for abdominal strengthener

Three Legged Dog to abdominal crunches

- Incorporate a leg and calf strength move by coming to the very tops of your toes on the inhale. As you exhale, lower your heels to the ground. Repeat as many times as desired. Continue to pull navel in towards the spine. Pull the inner groin into the pelvis.
- A core and chest strengthener is moving from Downward Facing Dog into Yoga Push up, with control. Repeat.
- Lift one leg, 3-Legged Dog, add a vinyasa flow from 3-Legged Dog to Push-Up or 3-Legged Dog to Warrior I, Warrior II, Reverse Warrior to High/Low Push Up.
- Knee and nose or elbow meet for a crunch.

To further progress...

REVOLVED DOWNWARD FACING DOG (PARIVRTTA ADHO MUKHA SVANASANA)

Getting into the Posture
1. Step feet in less than halfway towards palms.
2. Grasp the exterior ankle with opposite hand.

Counter Poses
- Table Top, Cat-Cow, Knees to Chest.
- Shoulder Stand, Headstand or Arm Balances.
- Forward Folds, Prone, or Supine back bends.

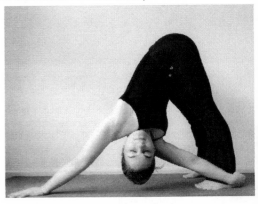

INVERSION POSTURES
EASY INVERSION / LEGS UP THE WALL (VIPARITA KARANI)

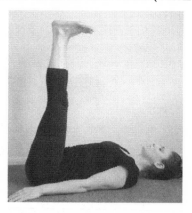

Each inhale brings restoration. Enjoy a new direction and a new perspective as you look above in this posture. Let each breath calm the mind chatter and rest the heart. Inhale gratitude and humility, exhale ego and prideful ways. Surrender everything to Him and rest in His promises. Rest my friend, in the arms of a loving God.

Getting into the Posture

1. Lying on your back, use a wall or simply extend your legs towards the sky.
2. Keep your spine long and skull on the ground.
3. May relax the feet for a restorative Legs up the Wall or engage the legs by pressing the heels up towards the sky. Use a blanket under the sacrum or neck if desired.

Modification

- Use a blanket under the shoulders and/or pelvis.
- Keep tailbone close to the wall; rest calves and heels on wall.
- Use a strap around the soles of the feet.
- Bend knees if needed (May also use a strap).

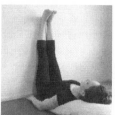 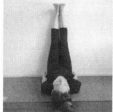

Use a pillow and/or wall

Deepen

- Open legs wide.
- Use a block under the shoulder blades to open the heart center.
- Do not use a wall; keep legs wide and engaged.

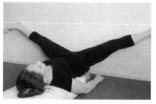

Open legs and/or block/pillow

PLOW POSE (HALASANA)

Release your old perspective. Inhale a fresh outlook. Continue to reach new depths in this pose. Inhale restoration and renewal, as you exhale any sickness and fatigue. Embrace new energy and vitality! God is your strength and your source!

Getting into the Posture
1. From Corpse Pose, using your core, gently come into Shoulder Stand preparation (Onto the broad part of the shoulders and place your hands on the lower back for support).
2. Extend your legs behind you so that your toes meet the ground or a prop at your chosen height.
3. Keep your gaze at the thighs; do not turn your head to either side in this posture.
4. Energetically lift the hamstrings towards the sky as you engage through the heels, pressing the feet behind you. Pull the navel in and upward.
5. Place the arms on the earth and engage.

Modification
- Do not come into full posture; place legs up the wall and enjoy a more restorative posture.
- Rest feet on blocks or a piece of furniture.
- Use a blanket under the shoulders and pelvis.
- Keep knees bent.

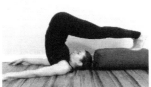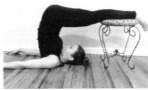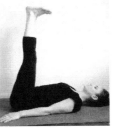

Use a tool of proper height

Stay in Legs Up The Wall

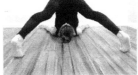

Wide Leg Plow

Deepen
- Continue to use each exhalation to walk the feet further back, releasing neck and upper back tension.
- Continue to broaden shoulder blades using resistance of arms, pressing the shoulder blades down and into the earth as you open the chest.
- Press through the heels energetically lifting the hamstrings towards the sky.
- Walk the hands back and clasp together.
- Practice Wide Leg Plow.

To further progress practice…

SIDE / REVOLVED PLOW (PARSVA HALASANA)

Getting into the Posture
1. From Wide Leg Plow, slide one foot over to the other; continue to press through the heels and lift through the hamstrings.
2. Practice keeping the hips high, directly above the shoulders some day.
3. Hold and switch sides.

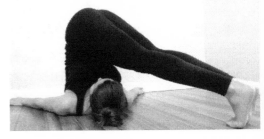

Deepening further, practice…

EAR PRESSURE POSE (KARNAPIDASANA)

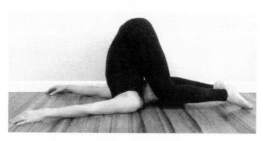

In this posture, feel the sensation of being calm, nurtured and safe. Listen to the sound of your heartbeat and breath. Meditate on gratitude for a healthy heart that beats with life and healing. Let your breath be calm, smooth and steady. Inhale safety and confidence as you exhale unhealthy isolation. Renew your hopes and dreams in this calming but energy-releasing posture.

Getting into the Posture
1. From Plow Pose, try to place the hips directly above the shoulders, supporting the lower back with both hands if needed.
2. Gently lower both knees to the ears and squeeze the ears to the head.
3. If possible, keep the tops of both feet on the earth.
4. Gently release, lowering down slowly, one vertebrae at a time.

Modification
- Do not come into full posture; practice Plow Pose or place legs up the wall and enjoy a restorative posture (Legs up the Wall).
- Rest knees on forehead or other prop, such as blocks on both side of the head.
- Use a blanket under the shoulders and pelvis.
- Tuck the toes under.
- Hands remain supporting your back.
- Practice Plow or Plow modifications.

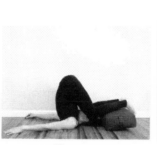
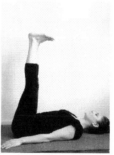

Use props   Legs Up The Wall

Deepen
- Continue to use each exhalation to walk the feet further back, releasing neck and upper back tension.
- Continue to broaden shoulder blades using resistance of arms, pressing the shoulder blades down and into the earth as you stretch the upper back.
- Press the knees into the ears.
- Walk the hands back and clasp together.
- Wrap arms around the back of knees and clasp opposite hand, wrist, or perhaps elbows.
- After wrapping arms around back of legs, clasp your hands under back of head, creating a pillow as you are in this intense but nurturing place.

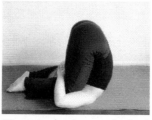

Wrap arms, hands rest on forehead

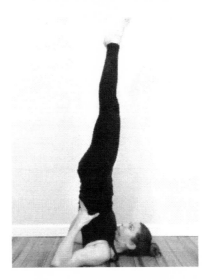

SHOULDER STAND (SARVANGASANA)

Inhale energy and new life here. Find your deepest expression of Shoulder Stand as you exhale tension and burdens that you are not meant to hold on to. Inhale a new vantage point and mind set as you exhale old programs and attitudes that no longer edify your life. Make the great exchange here, your heavy burdens and His light yoke!

Getting into the Posture
1. From Corpse Pose, bend the knees to extend the legs upward towards the sky.
2. Walk your arms behind your back as you extend them long; keep arms connected to the earth.
3. Using your core, lift upward and place the weight on the broad band of the shoulders; chin tucks in towards the chest.
4. Extend the legs straight and up. You may also come into other leg variations.
5. Do not turn your neck, keep the breath steady and calm.

Modification
- Do not come into full posture; practice Legs up the Wall and enjoy a restorative posture.
- Keep hands on small of back or hips to support.
- Use a blanket under the shoulders and pelvis.
- Practice Supported Shoulder Stand (Salamba Sarvangasana). Use the hands to support the lower back, keeping the elbows close to the body. Place a blanket under the broad of the shoulders if needed.

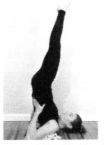

Supported Shoulder Stand

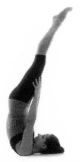

Deepen
- Continue to engage entire body and stretch throughout the neck and upper back.
- Explore leg variations.
- Advanced practitioners may practice Unsupported Shoulder Stand.

Unsupported Shoulder Stand

INVERSION POSTURES
HEADSTAND (SIRSASANA)

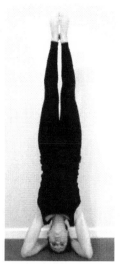

Inhale stability, balance and a renewed source of vitality. Exhale imbalances and "can't" out of your body, mind and spirit, as your entire system is being renewed. This is the "king" of all inversions and asanas; it will strengthen your entire being including your spirit. His strength is perfected in your weaknesses and His joy is your strength!

Getting into the Posture

1. From Dolphin pose, gently place the crown of your head on the earth, interlace all ten fingers behind the head, keeping the elbows close in.
2. Begin to walk your feet up towards the chest, while shifting the weight forward and allowing the forearms to "settle in" and bear the weight.
3. When you can no longer walk the feet in any further, bring both feet upward. If you bring one foot up at a time, be careful not to shift your weight extremely onto one side of the neck. Bringing both feet up at once will increase your strength for the full expression of Headstand.
4. Lengthen through the legs, engaging them inward as if you were standing in Mountain Pose.
5. Let the energy "sink down," allow your breath to be steady.

Modification

- Practice Legs up the Wall; use a wall for legs or feet.
- Practice Headstand against a wall.
- Practice Downward Facing Dog.
- Use a chair, similar prop, or a large exercise ball to drape yourself over to feel the sensation of being upside down. Try hanging your head off the edge of your bed, then move to hanging the torso off the edge.

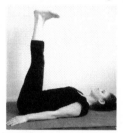

Legs Up The Wall

Deepen

- Continue to engage entire body while stretching throughout the neck and upper back.
- Practice various leg positions such as Half Lotus or Lotus legs.
- Try with no support of forearms, hands or wall, only the head (Only for experienced practitioners).

UNSUPPORTED HEADSTAND (NIRALAMBA SIRSASANA)

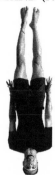

Only advanced practitioners should attempt this pose, as serious injury to the spinal cord and neck could occur. You must master Supported Headstand before attempting this posture. It is also a good idea to have assistance when getting into this pose. The entire body's weight is balanced on the head and the neck muscles.

Getting into the Posture

1. From Headstand, with caution, slowly move the arms in front of you as they lightly rest on the floor.
2. You will one day achieve the hands or arms bearing no weight at all and then progress to placing the arms by your sides or on the legs.

INVERSION POSTURES
TRIPOD HEADSTAND (SIRSASANA II)

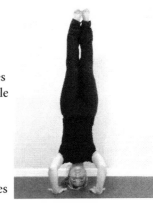

Getting into the Posture

1. From Wide A Frame Forward Fold, with fingers spread apart for a strong foundation, place your hands in front and center of torso.
2. Bring the crown of the head to the earth as you ensure your elbows are placed at the interior of the knees (The crown of your head and the palm of the hands create the "tripod or triangle" which serves as the stable foundation of this posture).
3. Your spine is elongated and torso is straightened before you lift the feet off the floor.
4. Come to the tops of the toes; use your core to extend your legs upward (Or practice any leg variation). Do not "dump" your weight into the shoulders.
5. Allow the weight to settle into the palms. Breath is calm and relaxed. Energy settles down.
6. Gently release in reverse order, as slowly as you achieved the posture. Your core strength brings your toes back down to Wide Leg Forward Fold. Release into a Half-Way Fold for a few breaths. Allow your sacrum to release safely before coming back to an upright position.

Practice leg variations:

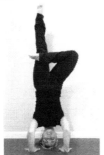 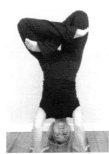 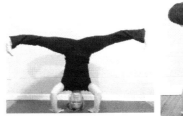 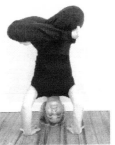

Tripod Headstands:
Half Lotus
Full Lotus
Wide Leg
Inverted Lotus

To deepen further, practice…

REVOLVED HEADSTAND (PARSVA SIRSASANA)

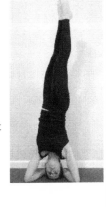

Continue to let your energy sink down towards the earth and settle into this posture. Embrace the energy and invigorating sensations as each inhale brings in new vision and clarity. Your exhalations will send out the old way of looking at things, the dead vision and dreams, as you continue to create space for new vision and dreams. With every exhalation, allow the twist to perhaps become deeper, allowing the Lord to breathe new life, energy and strength into you.

Getting into the Posture

1. From Headstand, turn your legs and torso away from each other. Remember that any revolved posture wrings out your organs as you twist and massage them. Adding the many twisting benefits to this deep inversion makes this a highly effective posture.

Deepen

- Continue to engage entire body and stretch throughout the neck and upper back.
- Practice various leg positions, Half or Full Lotus. Widen legs, bend legs forward and backward.
- Come into Sideways Hero Pose by bending both knees; heels contact buttocks as you are twisting.

To further progress, practice…

UPWARD / INVERTED STAFF (URDHVA DANDASANA)

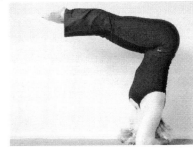

Getting into the Posture

1. From Headstand, engage the core as you strengthen your posture.
2. Slowly begin to lower the legs so they become parallel to the earth. Feet are flexed or relaxed.
3. Slowly release the legs to the ground when you're ready.

INVERSION POSTURES
FULL ARM BALANCE / HANDSTAND (ADHO MUKHA VRKSASANA)

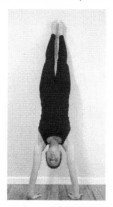

Getting into the Posture

1. From Downward Facing Dog, walk your feet towards your head as much as possible.
2. Lifting to the tops of the toes, let the weight settle into the upper body and hands (Fingers spread apart for a strong foundation). Experiment with fingers directly forward, or facing slightly out to the side, see which one feels more stable.
3. Using your core strength, (think of "zipping up the rib cage") bring your knees toward your torso then extend the legs upward. If you bring one foot up at a time, be careful to not shift your weight extremely onto one side of the neck. Bringing both feet up at once will increase your strength for the full expression of Handstand. Do not "dump your weight" into the shoulders. Create space between the ears and shoulders. The goal is to be completely vertical, as if you were standing in Mountain Pose.
4. Gaze is neutral to the spine (Slightly forward and down).

Embrace this challenge of mind over fear. Inhale confidence and patience. Exhale insecurities and frustrations. As you continue your journey into your deepest expression of this posture, surrender to the unknown and embrace it. Trust in Him at all times.

Also practice...

ONE HANDED ARM BALANCE (EKA HASTA VRKSASANA)

For advanced practitioners only. Master Handstand before attempting this posture.

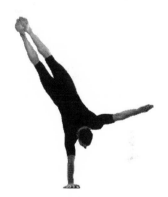

Getting into the Posture

1. Allow your energy to settle into your Handstand.
2. Gripping the earth with one hand and using the core strength to remain strong in posture and alignment, cautiously lift the other hand off the earth.
3. Breathe! Remain sturdy and steadfast.

Though You have made me see troubles, many and bitter, You will restore my life again; from the depths of the earth You will again bring me up. Psalm 71:20

Prayer:
Thank you, Father, for making all things new! Whenever I doubt You, have fears or anxiety, I can get upside down and You will speak into me a NEW perspective with a new "take" on my circumstance. Thank You for ears to hear and eyes to see You, no matter what I face or the position I am in. I will praise You at ALL times. Praises for You will continually be in my mouth!

FLOWING IN GRACE

The more we spend time with others the more we get to know them. We get to know what brings them joy and sadness we see their faults and character flaws. The time we invest in others allows us to experience a deeper, intimate connection with them. It's important to protect our inner circle and travel with people who are heading in the same direction as us. Our relationships influence us and can have a profound effect, positively or negatively, upon our lives.

What would happen if you got into the habit of spending more time with God? Spending time with Him and seeking Him would allow you to know Him more intimately. The great news about God is that He has no faults or character flaws. Anything that "rubs off" on you can *only* be amazing!

As we grow in Christ, His ways and heart begin to influence everything in our lives. As we begin to know the heart of God, we understand the things that hurt His heart, as well as the things that make Him smile. In turn, these things will bring us joy or sorrow. I often pray, "Lord, give me a burden for lost souls." Well, this prayer did not come from my fleshly heart. It came from spending time with my Father. His heart eventually became *my* heart's cry. When we get saved, we become one with Him. His spirit resides inside us and we are intimately one. We can pray silently and He will hear our prayers even if we do not speak them. He actually knows the thought before it was perceived. We don't have to scream, shout and hope that our prayers make it to Heaven. No, He is inside us; He hears our prayers and thoughts before they even occur.

When we are intimate with God and the Holy Spirit, we get into a "sweet spot." We flow in His grace. Our prayers are *set in motion*. We communicate constantly, even laugh together. Hidden mysteries and treasures are revealed. There are no secrets in the secret place. We just have to get there. Throughout scripture, we learn that we have to "go" first. We seek first. We knock first. We draw near first. Then we find Him. He opens the door, and then He draws nearer to us.

Draw near to God and He will draw near to you. James 4:8

In this incredible sweet spot, grace washes over us. His grace is always greater and always sufficient. All you have to do is simply receive it.

From His abundance we have all received one gracious blessing after another! John 1:16

Take note. We have *already received* these gracious blessings, one after another. Can you picture it? Imagine yourself flowing in God's great grace, moving in and out of His love and embrace. Can you see yourself *completely enveloped* in His presence? Now picture this presence gone. It can be a scary thought. We can do nothing without Him and as soon as we are no longer enveloped in His presence, darkness creeps in. I encourage you to stay in the *dance of grace* with your Heavenly Father. He will guide, and all you have to do is follow and trust. That is all you [ever] have to "do." We serve a mighty God, don't we? It is simple to receive this abundant life. Believe, trust and follow. That is it! Why do we want to complicate what He has already given us? We have *already* received all of His blessings. We certainly do not deserve it. Are you overjoyed that we do not get what we deserve? Why are we so stingy as Christians with extending grace, mercy and forgiveness to others? We should freely extend what we have so freely been given. We can get a little holier-than-thou when it comes to extending something that we think someone does not deserve. Well, all we have to ask ourselves is, "Did I deserve the forgiveness, love, grace and blessings that the Lord has so freely given to me?"

Great grace! Stay in the flow of His grace.

Remember the flow of grace as you practice praying in motion. YogaFaith is, quite literally, your prayers in motion. Dancing in grace. Flowing in grace and worshiping the One who has blessed you exceedingly and abundantly - more than you could ever imagine!

In yoga, the word Vinyasa is defined as *continuous movement*. You are flowing with your breath. In YogaFaith, knowing the One Who gives us breath and setting our intentions on the Lord allows our flow, or continuous movement in prayer, to become transformational.

There are numerous postures and poses in yoga. Linking them together and moving in and out of postures is known as Vinyasa Flow. You can follow a preset flow, or create your own based on your personal needs. You can practice a slow, gentle flow, or an energizing and powerful flow. If you are sore or lethargic, you may focus on more of a stretching or restorative flow. If you need energy or balance, you can practice inversions, back bends and balancing postures in your flow. You can create your own amazing and fun routines, perhaps to different worship songs. I call this "YogaFaith Dance!" It is amazing to have a playlist ready to go at any given time. You can push play on your "healing" playlist. Need rest? Just push play and receive His peaceful rest. Perhaps one day you need energy. Your powerful praise and worship music will guide you into an amazing flow with the Almighty! Be safe, and put sequences together that make sense so you do not compromise alignment or joints. This is a time to be creative and be with the Lord in many different ways of worship. God loves variety. If you fixed meatloaf every night your family would get bored. I believe that God loves to see us worship and spend time with Him in new, fun and creative ways. Get your family and friends involved. Set aside one night a week where you and your spouse or family get together and connect in this powerful way of making God the center of your family and home.

A standard Vinyasa Flow that you may have already experienced if you practice yoga, is Sun Salutation A and Sun Salutation B. In YogaFaith we refer to them as "Son" Salutations. They are a routine or sequence, designed to energize the body and create internal heat (think of stoking a fire). Generally, each movement is given one part of the breath. You want to enjoy the transitions of flowing just as much as you enjoy the postures themselves.

Son Salutations can be your entire practice, or they can be woven into a practice. If you are new to yoga, be patient with yourself while learning the basic poses. Establish breath control, good alignment, and then move into the Son Salutations. You may also modify or alter the sequences; there are no rules here, just freedom. I encourage you to step out of the box, not just during a Son Saluta-tion, but also in life. Explore and become a blessing to others with your own unique and God-given talents.

SON SALUTATION A

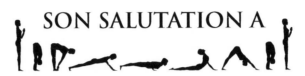

1. Mountain Pose – Inhale
2. Standing Forward Fold – Exhale
3. Lift halfway up – Inhale
4. Plank Pose – Exhale & Inhale
5. Yoga Push up – Exhale
6. Cobra/Upward Facing Dog – Inhale
7. Downward Facing Dog – Exhale and breathe 3-5 breaths
8. Step (or leap) both feet forward to Standing, Forward Fold – Exhale
9. Sweep arms up to Mountain – Inhale
10. Repeat if you desire

SON SALUTATION B

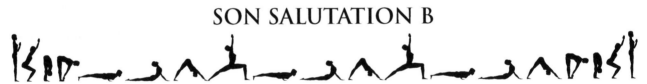

1. Mountain Pose – Inhale
2. Chair Pose – Exhale/Inhale
3. Standing Forward Fold – Exhale
4. Lift halfway up – Inhale
5. Yoga Push up – Exhale
6. Cobra/Upward Facing Dog – Inhale
7. Downward Facing Dog – Exhale and breathe 3-5 breaths
8. Right foot Warrior 1 – Inhale
9. Yoga Push Up – Exhale
10. Cobra/Upward Facing Dog – Inhale
11. Downward Facing Dog – Exhale
12. Left foot Warrior 1 – Inhale
13. Yoga Push Up – Exhale
14. Cobra/Upward Facing Dog – Inhale
15. Downward Facing Dog – Exhale and breathe 3-5 breaths
16. Step both feet forward to Standing Forward Fold – Exhale
17. Lift halfway up – Inhale
18. Chair Pose – Inhale/ Exhale
19. Mountain Pose – Inhale/Exhale

MEDITATIONS FOR SON SALUTATION

FOCUS ON THE REAL SON AS YOU PRACTICE SON SALUTATION A

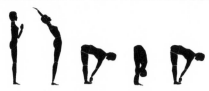

Our Father, who art in Heaven, [inhale arms rise] *hallowed be Thy name* [exhale Forward Fold].
Your kingdom come, Your will be done [inhale up to Half Forward Fold],
on Earth as it is in Heaven.

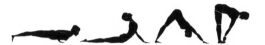

[walk or float back, exhale to the bottom of a push up] *Give us this day our daily bread,* [inhale to Cobra or Upward Facing Dog]
and forgive us our sins, as we have forgiven those who sin against us, [exhale back to Downward Facing Dog]
And lead us not into temptation, and deliver us from all evil, [inhale to Half Forward Fold]

[exhale Forward Fold] *For Yours is the kingdom,* [inhale Upward Salute] *and the power and the glory forever*
[return to Mountain] *Amen.*
Matthew 6:9-13

The Greatest Commandment - Mark 12:28-31
One of the teachers of the law came and heard them debating. Noticing that Jesus had given them a good answer, he asked Him, "Of all the commandments, which is the most important?" Jesus answered, "The foremost is, 'HEAR, O ISRAEL! THE LORD OUR GOD IS ONE LORD AND YOU SHALL LOVE THE LORD YOUR GOD WITH ALL YOUR HEART, AND WITH ALL YOUR SOUL, AND WITH ALL YOUR MIND, AND WITH ALL YOUR STRENGTH. "The second is this, 'YOU SHALL LOVE YOUR NEIGHBOR AS YOURSELF.' There is no other commandment greater than these..."

YogaFaith was birthed through Mark 12:30 to worship with *our whole being.* As you meditate on the greatest two commandments, to love God and your neighbor, you can choose to sit in stillness or flow with one of the Son Salutations. Keep in mind the powerful and miraculous being that you are. With this particular Son Salutation, combined with Mark 12:28-31, worship your Creator as you never have before, with your whole spirit, heart, soul and physical body.

DIG IN THE WORD. YOUR SOUL WORK; MARK 12
A MEDITATION FOR SON SALUTATIONS

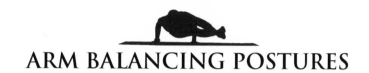

ARM BALANCING POSTURES

Our Lord is great and rich in power; His understanding has no limitation.
Psalm 147:5 International Standard Version

HIS STRENGTH > MY WEAKNESSES

And He has said to me, "My grace is sufficient for you, for my power is perfected in weakness."
Most gladly, therefore, I will rather boast about my weaknesses,
so that the power of Christ may dwell in me. 2 Corinthians 12:9 English Standard Version

I would rather boast about my weaknesses, so that His power would dwell in me. Wow! Is this the opposite of our fleshly, natural selves? His strength is perfected in our weakness.

There have been many times in my life when this verse has had to consume me. There have been times when I wanted to give in and give up. In 2004, I wanted to give up on everything. After losing my job, my marriage and almost losing my home, I thought I had lost everything. I was consumed with depression, discouragement and hopelessness. At the time, I didn't see any way out of the darkness except to check out, of life. I remember looking at a closet full of clothes, and thinking, "There will never be a reason to get dressed up ever again." I thought to myself, it was the whispers of the enemy, that I would never laugh or feel joy again. There were days when my mother called me – and I can still hear her voice – and said, "Mish, you have to get up and open the blinds. Please *let some light in.*" Yes, I was in complete and utter darkness. I could barely get up to feed my two dogs. Thank God I didn't have children to care for. I finally made the gut-wrenching decision to take my own life.

I decided how and where I would kill myself. I decided that swallowing pills would be the easiest route. I would do it in the master bedroom of my home in North Portland. As I opened the closet doors in my bedroom, the Lord spoke audibly to me. His voice, a still, small whisper said, "By doing this, you will kill your own mother of a broken heart." For the first time in months, I instantly came to my senses. In one millisecond, self-pity dissolved, and my thoughts became slightly more rational. The thought of killing my own mother sent shock waves to my heart. I didn't know when, why, or how, but I knew taking my own life was not the answer. It would be the most selfish act I could ever commit. Besides, I would have killed the wrong girl – literally!

It was not easy to move forward. I had to do the work, and it was a lot of work! It was a long uphill road and I fought many battles and demons along the way. But today, I am so far removed from the girl that I am speaking about, that it is as if I am talking about a stranger. He made something so beautiful out of something so dark and ugly. The Lord could not have turned my ashes into something so beautiful had I not been willing to surrender them in the first place. (See Isaiah 61:3) The devil is the father of all lies! I decided to trust the Lord with my life. I was humbled to the point that all I could do was get on my knees and surrender. I remember opening the book of Psalm and letting out a whisper of a voice to read these passages out loud. The Holy Spirit was telling me to put voice to the scripture, and although I did not feel like speaking, I did. What started out as a whisper of the scriptures eventually turned into shouting, claiming and declaring His promises. By the end of the year, I was shouting at the devil and speaking my world into existence by putting voice to God's promises. I began to see His promises and handiwork manifest before my very eyes!

The Lord's strength was absolutely perfected in all my weaknesses! His promise of restoring double for my trouble came true. To be honest, in the beginning of my uphill battle, it was not absolute trust. It was almost wishing, crossing my fingers and hoping as I read His promises out loud that they *might* come to pass. But as I began to see miracles manifest by speaking my world into existence, I began to realize that His promises are true. They are yes and Amen! His promises do not come back void. Isaiah 55:11 is something that I have seen come to pass and so can you....*so is My word that goes out from my mouth: It will not return to me empty, but will accomplish what I desire and achieve the purpose for which I sent it.*

As you have probably gathered, I love The Message bible. This is how 2 Corinthians 12:7-10 reads. It is eloquently written and sums up my days of darkness. May these words encourage you in your times of weakness and darkness.

Because of the extravagance of those revelations, and so I wouldn't get a big head,
I was given the gift of a handicap to keep me in constant touch with my limitations.
Satan's angel did his best to get me down; what he in fact did was push me to my knees.
No danger then of walking around high and mighty!
At first I didn't think of it as a gift, and begged God to remove it. Three times I did that, and then He told me,
"My grace is enough; it's all you need. My strength comes into its own in your weakness."
Once I heard that, I was glad to let it happen. I quit focusing on the handicap and began appreciating the gift. It was a case of Christ's strength moving in on my weakness. Now I take limitations in stride, and with good cheer, these limitations that cut me down to size—abuse, accidents, opposition, bad breaks. I just let Christ take over! And so the weaker I get, the stronger I become.
2 Corinthians 12:7-10 The Message

To say the least, I was humbled. It was a much-needed humbling. I love *The Message*. It reads: "What he in fact did was push me to my knees." What the devil meant as harm towards me, God used for my good! It was on my knees that I truly encountered Christ.

ARM BALANCING POSTURES

During my divorce and the process of losing everything, the enemy had me deceived. I had a narrow perspective and was living a self-centered life based on this deception. The things I thought would make me happy were just a facade; the enemy painted a bright and beautiful picture to make these things attractive. I fell for his tricks, hook, line and sinker. In the end, satan ever-so-gently tapped me on my shoulder and whispered, "I lied." My life was blown up because I was deceived. The devil is a liar! He is the god of this world. We cannot be a friend of God and a friend to this world. We must choose. Everyday we have choices. The most important decision you must make every day of your life is to choose life! Choose joy. Choose peace, even though storms may be all around you. Choose to live for God, obedient to His word, and He will reward you with joy and peace unspeakable. His promise to you is a life of abundance, not barely getting by, sad and depressed. He promises a life of fullness, wholeness, and eternal life, far beyond this world has ever known or our imaginations could ever dream of.

My then-husband had wanted to stay together, but I made the difficult decision *not* to stay married. When I was divorced, fired from my long-time job, and alone, the enemy had his way in my mind and heart. I thought I would even lose my house, which sits only a few blocks from my mother's house where I grew up. I loved having my mom so close. My home was, well, my home; the thought of losing it devastated me. I worked in the stone industry for almost 20 years. I had remodeled the home I shared with my husband with all my favorite stones: granites, travertine, slate and onyx; it was my sanctuary. Even though I wanted to keep the house, I was alone. Just what I wanted, right? I used to tell God that I couldn't wait for it to be five years down the road because *surely* in five years, this season would have passed. I knew if I could make it out of this pit, in five years I would most likely be happy again.

The Lord is my redeemer! He even prospers all my mistakes! Isn't this amazing? Do you know that to this day, I still own that gem of a house in North Portland? God has blessed me with great tenants throughout the years and protected the property that I fell in love with so long ago. After losing everything once again years later, sometimes the rent from this home was the only income I had. Remember when I told you my reading and praying out loud was sometimes wishing and hoping? I used to say, "Thank you, Father, that my life looks unrecognizable! Thank You for prospering my mistakes. I am truly forgiven and set free! Thank You for always providing for me. Thank You for perfecting everything that concerns me! (Psalm 138:8) I praise You for being my Jehovah Nissi, my victory and protection! I thank You for being my Jehovah Jireh, the provider of my every single need. I never go without; nothing is missing, broken or lacking in my life! I am redeemed; I am made righteous through the precious blood of the Lamb!" I would walk through my whole house declaring these promises and believing each one of them as if they had *already* happened. That's because in the spiritual and eternal realm, they already had happened. You see, we must speak our life into existence! Every day, we have the power to choose: life or death, life-giving words, or words of death. The choice is always ours.

Well, obviously, I'm still alive for such a time as this. God has a plan for each of us. His plans are for your good and He will never harm you! (Jeremiah 29:11) The key is to surrender those ashes for beauty. God can never do anything with your ashes until you surrender them to Him. You must invite Him into to those innermost parts and let Him heal, cleanse and restore your ashes. It is time to exchange beauty for those ashes and receive His garment of praise. Step out of the old garments and put on something brand new! He will turn your mourning into dancing, I promise! (See Isaiah 61)

In 2014, I celebrated the tenth anniversary of not taking my life! Even though I told myself I would never get married again, God had other plans. He blessed me with an amazing husband, someone I grew up with. We constantly bumped into each other, and one day, he asked me out to dinner. It was August 2007. He purchased a ring in October, and we were married in March 2008. In June 2008, we embarked on a new venture with a few business partners and moved to Washington State. As my husband toiled away at our new business, I attempted to go back to work in the stone industry, but it was like going back to Egypt. I was in a car accident while working one day and was let go due to the accident. It was a blessing in disguise, but I felt lost and tossed among the waves of the ocean. Once again, I didn't know what to do. God soon confirmed to me that what I'd been trying to accomplish in my own strength was yesterday. That season has passed and He wanted me to do something new.

See, I am doing a new thing! Now it springs up; do you not perceive it? I am making a way in the wilderness and streams in the wasteland.
Isaiah 43:19

I didn't want to miss this "new thing" God was going to do. Before He did it, I tried things in my own strength. I tried a few mediocre jobs, but felt lost and confused about my purpose. It was another frustrating season of often asking and desperately pleading with Him, "What, God? What is it? Where do You want me? What do You want me to do?" I was lost, trying to find my way, while my husband and our business partners plowed away at laying a new foundation for a brand-new, multiple-location franchise.

While I was trying to find my way, I saw many red flags about our partners in business. We had uprooted our entire lives and invested all we had for this business adventure. Recently married, we'd both quit our long-term, financially-stable careers, and left our friends, family, colleagues and support systems back in Oregon where we had been rooted our entire lives. My husband had owned a successful business for more than a decade. I'd had a secure, high-paying career in the design field for almost 20 years. We were comfortable and financially secure, with lots of cushion in the bank and investments. After my husband sold his profitable company, individually we rolled everything we had into our new adventure. After much hard work, trust, faith, blood, sweat, and tears, our "business partners" squandered all of our invested money blindly from under us. We lost everything.

ARM BALANCING POSTURES

One day when I believed only what I could *see*, I was confident we were going to lose our house. Forgetting again what I needed to do, I called my mom. She reminded me to plead the blood of Jesus over my front and back door and remind the devil that he was trespassing. It was one of those movie moments, you know, the one where you hang up and find yourself sliding down the wall to cry. I cried. I was cowering with my back against the front door, weeping. Then I heeded my mother's words, stirred myself up, turned around and laid hands on our front door to declare boldly, "satan, you cannot have this home! I plead the blood of Jesus over this home and our lives; we are protected and we will STAY in Jesus' name!" As I write these lines, sitting not too far from that same front door, I am overwhelmed with the protection, provision and faithfulness of our God. When we think we have lost it all, we only gain something far richer than we can imagine. We gain trust, faith and intimacy with the all-knowing, all-faithful, Living God. As Sue Monk Kidd describes, "Crisis is a summons into transformation." (*When the Heart Waits*, by Sue Monk Kidd)

Nothing creates more intimacy with Christ than fasting and praying. I practice the Daniel fast, a practice based on the fasting principles of the Prophet Daniel, at the beginning of each year. One January during one of these fasts, the Lord called me to share His love and healing through yoga. I had enjoyed the practice and study of yoga since the late eighties while dancing, but I never dreamed of becoming a yoga teacher. I could dance in front of thousands at large stadiums, but I could *never* speak in front of people. So I thought. Remember, the devil is a liar. Thankfully, our thoughts are not God's thoughts. He tells us to go into the world and preach the gospel, heal the sick and much more. Well, this requires speaking to others, often large crowds.

Out of obedience, I established YogaFaith. YogaFaith is not only a safe place for Christians to practice yoga, but also a place that others will connect with Christ; perhaps meet Him for the first time. It is also a community and family doing life together. Here, non-believers have a chance to encounter a living God on a yoga mat. You do not have to be a Christian to practice YogaFaith. It is all-inclusive, never exclusive. You are invited to come as you are, no matter who you are, what you believe or don't believe. It is simply a time to surrender and let go of things that entangle us. My prayer is that people simply leave changed and more whole.

YogaFaith is first about Jesus and secondly about yoga. YogaFaith offers classes, workshops, retreats and teacher trainings. It is one of the only Christian academies accredited and recognized by the Yoga Alliance, an international nonprofit that sets guidelines and standards for becoming an internationally recognized yoga trainer. We offer teacher training programs throughout the world to certify others in sharing the good news of Christ and to guide others into the God-given gift of yoga. It is truly a life-changing and transformational program. I would have never dreamed it possible. After getting alone with Christ, emptying myself out so that I could hear from Him, He blessed me with a powerful gift and message. No matter what we are doing in our everyday lives, we are to glorify Him. God certainly chose the "least of them" to bless others with this ministry.

It hasn't always been easy. When you step out in obedience to the Lord, remember that He doesn't promise comfort or convenience. "Christians" may be the first to attack what God speaks into you. Friends and family may leave you, but trust in the Lord; He has it all planned out. The thing about YogaFaith is that some Christians have a problem with yoga while some yogis have issues with Jesus. That is okay, because what others think about you, YogaFaith, or me is none of our business. We need to know who we are in Christ and, more importantly, we need to know what He has called us to do. He called *me* to YogaFaith and the day YogaFaith becomes about anything else but Him, I don't want it. It isn't up to me to absorb others' judgment or opinions. You actually would have to *experience* YogaFaith before you can speak about it. Remember the definition of yoga is *to yoke*, and the definition of faith is *belief in things you cannot see*. My only defense of YogaFaith is the Name above all names; it's all about Jesus! He is the center of everything! Jesus Himself did not defend His innocence and righteousness when people (including religious and authoritative leaders) attacked Him. The same is true for you and me. We cannot defend Jesus.

So, God gave me a dream, but this dream required *faith*. And this faith required *action*. There were many times when I questioned God. During an intense and difficult pruning season, one day as I drove from Portland to Seattle, I asked Him again, "Are You sure? Is this from You? Is this what You want me to do?" He answered swiftly, "Yes. Now, do not ask again."

From that day forward, I had complete trust in God's call for my life. I put my all into this ministry. YogaFaith might not be my final destination but He led me to it for such a time as now. Because He supernaturally blessed it, there is no question that YogaFaith is a gift from God. Do not question in darkness what the Lord has spoken to you in light. In the beginning of anything, we start with a lot of excitement, passion and enthusiasm. But this can quickly dissipate as we begin the journey towards our dream. Passion and excitement cannot and will not keep you on the path, but your character, tenacity, trust in God and perseverance will carry you over the finish line.

Now, I am enjoying what I always searched for: The "sweet spot." You know, that thing you hear about and then say, "Lord, I want that!" I heard other people saying they were in their "sweet spot," and I always imagined what that must feel like. Today, I am here to tell you that it is all possible. You already know this if you know Matthew 19:26, *With man this is impossible, but with God all things are possible.*

DO NOT QUESTION IN DARKNESS WHAT THE LORD HAS SPOKEN TO YOU IN LIGHT
V. Raymond Edman

ARM BALANCING POSTURES

What I want to share with you today is that you must listen to the Lord. Do not listen to those around you, even if it is a family member. Protect your inner circle and surround yourself with those that support and edify you. Find good mentors and people that will greatly influence you and bring you *up*, so that you can grow your dream with God and the people He sends you in life for your journey. It is much like an airplane. Be wise in choosing the people you will travel with and make sure they are going to the same destination.

As a Kingdom builder, you are on the front line of any battle. The attacks come, sometimes so much that it seems in the natural that they will overtake you. You should expect battles. You should *prepare* for battles in the innermost secret place so that you can stand strong and be victorious in the outer courts. You want to ensure you are always dressed for battle, armed and protected. You should also know that there will be times of great loneliness, where God will prune and shake everything that no longer serves your destiny. I can only say, "Trust God; always lean on Him and allow *Him* to fight for you."

You will not have to fight this battle. Take up your positions; stand firm and see the deliverance the Lord will give you, Judah and Jerusalem. Do not be afraid; do not be discouraged. Go out to face them tomorrow, and the Lord will be with you. 2 Chronicles 20:17

Praying for those who attack you will help you through it; I promise. It doesn't start out easy. Then the Lord changes your heart and it actually becomes enjoyable. You will never be so transformed than when you pray for your enemies! This is what the Lord spoke to Jehoshaphat as he went to battle;

Do not be afraid or discouraged because of this vast army. For the battle is not yours, but God's. Tomorrow march down against them. They will be climbing up by the Pass of Ziz, and you will find them at the end of the gorge in the Desert of Jeruel. You will not have to fight this battle. Take up your positions; stand firm and see the deliverance the Lord will give you, Judah and Jerusalem. Do not be afraid; do not be discouraged. Go out to face them tomorrow, and the Lord will be with you." 2 Chronicles 20:15-17

In the natural realm, Jehoshaphat looked around at the sheer number of enemies that surrounded him and his small army. But, we do not serve a natural God! The Lord did a mighty work this day. Verse 20 says:
As they began to sing and praise, the Lord set ambushes against the men.

God is saying to you and me today what He said so many years ago to Jehoshaphat. Be still. The battle is not yours; you will not have to fight, only stand firm to see God deliver you. *When* you praise Him, He takes care of *everything* and will *immediately* set up ambushes against your enemies. Wow! I encourage you to read the entire passage of Second Chronicles 20. During my darkest hours in 2004, while reading the Bible through in the following year, this one passage changed all my darkness and brought me into the light. It is imprinted on my heart and I call on it during any attack.

I have gone from the trenches of dark despair to the light of His glory. He continues to take me from glory to glory to glory. I share my story and speak to people who are going through divorce, depression and other heavy burdens that we sometimes think we have to carry on our own. Our tests are our testimonies. Without your mess, you do not have a message. So count it *all* glory. And never let the enemy shut your mouth. Your story can help someone; it could save someone's life. You can give hope where there is no hope. I was ashamed of my darkest hours. Depression, suicide, divorce, addictions, and some other things not mentioned, are not always subjects we feel comfortable discussing. I promise you that the enemy would like nothing more than for you to feel ashamed, condemned and embarrassed. However, the reason we are alive is to help others. Do not remain silent. I double-dog dare you to stop living in fear, start using your strengths and your messes for the glory of God.

Consider it pure joy, my brothers and sisters, whenever you face trials of many kinds, because you know that the testing of your faith produces perseverance. Let perseverance finish its work so that you may be mature and complete, not lacking anything. If any of you lacks wisdom, you should ask God, who gives generously to all without finding fault, and it will be given to you. But when you ask, you must believe and not doubt, because the one who doubts is like a wave of the sea, blown and tossed by the wind. That person should not expect to receive anything from the Lord. Such a person is double-minded and unstable in all they do. James 1:2-8

Whether you are fighting for your life or fighting for your dream, it will take hard work, perseverance, strength, determination and complete trust in the Lord.

This is a great introduction to what can sometimes be a very challenging asana family. Arm Balancing postures require all of these: strength, determination and trust. You must stay committed and determined if you want to achieve some of these postures; they won't always come easily. Remember, His strength is perfected in your weakness!

ARM BALANCING POSTURES

The Lord God is my strength, He has made my feet like hinds' feet,
and makes me walk on my high places. Habakkuk 3:19

The Lord is my strength and my shield; my heart trusts in Him, and I am helped: therefore my heart greatly rejoices; and with my song will
I praise Him. The Lord is their strength, and He is the saving strength of His anointed.
Save your people, and bless your inheritance: feed them also, and lift them up forever. Psalm 28:7-9

Arm balancing postures require great strength; trust in the Lord and yourself. The journey of mastering any balancing posture demands much patience. This is especially true for arm balances. You may need to remind yourself, "Hang in there," or "Embrace the journey," or "Worship while I wait," or "I put my trust in Him," or, "I am becoming stronger and stronger." The more you practice, the stronger you will become and the closer you will get to mastering arm balancing postures. Transformation always requires process. Trust the process.

Any balancing posture will strengthen reflexes and help in preventing injuries. The lack of challenging our muscles and bones as we age contributes to loss of mineralization in bones, which could lead to osteoporosis and other muscle-joint issues. Balancing postures will aid in preventing osteoporosis as well as build entire body strength and overall confidence. Proper awareness of alignment and engagement must be present when practicing any balancing posture.

A great place to begin with arm balancing postures is in Plank or Downward Facing Dog, as there is moderate weight distributed through the arms and shoulders. As you strengthen the upper body, you can begin to practice more challenging arm balancing postures. Don't be afraid of arm balances; embrace the journey. As you would when learning any asana family, be patient as you strengthen the muscles needed. These may begin as difficult poses but just like anything, the more you practice the more you develop strength and the better you will become.

TRANSFORMATION ALWAYS REQUIRES PROCESS

Begin practicing with blocks to elevate the floor closer to you. You may also want to start on a carpeted or cushioned floor. As the blocks will aid in the postures, you can note how the posture feels and what it requires. Once you understand the mechanisms of the pose, then you can progress in the posture without the use of blocks or other props.

Benefits of arm balancing postures include, but are not limited to:
- Strengthens the entire body, specifically chest, wrists, arms, shoulders, neck, thighs, hamstrings, buttocks and the entire core center.
- Improves alignment of the spine, improving posture and increasing mobility of spine.
- Stretches and opens the neck, chest, lungs, shoulders and abdominal.
- Strengthens and stimulates every bodily system, specifically the respiratory, cardiovascular and endocrine systems.
- Stretches throat, stimulates thyroid and parathyroid glands, improving metabolism.
- Stimulates digestion and aids in circulation.
- Can be therapeutic for mild cases of asthma, osteoporosis, carpal tunnel and sinusitis.
- Relieves constipation, menstrual discomfort and menopause symptoms.
- Increases stamina, energizes and rejuvenates.
- Improves concentration, focus, mental clarity, balance, strength and energy.
- Relieves stress, anxiety and depression.
- Renewing, strengthening and revitalizing.

Cautions include, but are not limited to:
- Serious wrist, back, neck or shoulder injury.
- High or low blood pressure, other heart problems.
- Severe sinusitis, insomnia, glaucoma, diarrhea, asthma, vertigo, pregnancy or carpal tunnel.
- If you have a headache, high or low blood pressure, diabetes or other heart issues, practice modifications or avoid some postures.

Remember to rely on the Lord during this asana family. Surrender your fears, doubts and weaknesses to Him. Allow His *perfect* strength to take over and then trust Him *completely*. Even if you fall, the key is to get up and try again. I often say in classes, "If you fall [in an arm balance], the floor isn't that far away!" Just as in our darkest hours, we have to keep pressing forward. We have to place one foot in front of the other, take one day at a time and keep moving.

Keep at it and like most anything else in life, the hard work will be worth it. God will always use our mess for a message. It is the very reason you still have a heartbeat. You friend, were created to glorify God. Don't allow the enemy to shut your mouth and keep you in shame, guilt and condemnation. Share your story; share your God.

Prayer:

Thank you, Father, for giving me a newfound boldness and confidence in You! I am strong IN You and I'm able to do all things through You. Forgive me for listening to the lies of the enemy. I want to live for You and allow my mess to glorify You and bless others. You bringing me through all my junk has prepared me to help many people! I know that You will make a way for me to help them. Your Spirit will always give me the right words to say and speak to me about the direction I need to follow. Thank You, Lord, for confidence in You! Thank you for Your strength that fights my battles when I move out of the way for You to do so! Thank You for wisdom, joy, peace and the ability to be still so that I can continue to hear the many important things You want to speak into me. I praise You for fearfully and wonderfully creating me and I know that You have predestined my days to be glorious and abundant. I am so grateful to You for revealing hidden mysteries and treasures so great! I smile at my future and cannot wait to see what the windows of Heaven will drop in my spirit! I am excited to share the Good News with those around me. I will no longer shut my mouth, but will glorify all that You have done in my life. I will tell all who will hear that You are the reason for my joy and my victory! With every breath that I have Lord, may every inhale and every exhale magnify and glorify You! Amen and Amen, glory to the King of Kings, the Prince of Peace and the Name that is above all names!

GOD WILL ALWAYS USE YOUR MESS FOR A MESSAGE

DIG IN THE WORD. YOUR SOUL WORK; ISAIAH 40, A MEDITATION FOR ARM BALANCES

THE POSTURES

STRETCHING TIGER POSE (VYAGHRASANA)

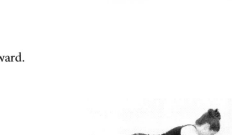

Every inhalation brings in expansion. Broaden your horizon and perspective. Outstretch your limbs and lengthen your capacity to receive. As you exhale, send out anything that no longer aligns with the will of God. Receive all that He has for you. Accept it, and then secure those things closest to you.

Preparatory Poses
- Table Top
- Cat-Cow
- Seated Twist
- Forward Folding Poses

Getting into the Posture
1. Kneeling in Table Top pose, extend one leg out behind you keeping the hips squared forward.
2. Extend the opposite arm out, reaching through all five fingers.
3. Engage the core. Hold the posture, or add strengthening moves such as crunches.

Modification
- Stay in Table Top.
- Only extend the leg or the arm, not both at the same time.
- Come down to your forearms and focus only on the leg.
- Coming into a supine position and practice sit-ups.

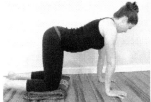

Use a blanket

Deepen
- Energetically hug every muscle to every bone as you come into your deepest expression.
- Let your exhalations bring the elbow and knee to connect midline as you tuck your chin into your chest, also massaging the thyroid and parathyroid glands, which stimulates the metabolism, and flow through the crunches.
- You may also practice Tiger/Half Tiger in Vinyasa with Low Lunge, Pigeon, or Abdominal Crunches as mentioned above.

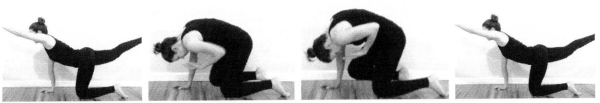

Stretching Tiger with abdominal crunches

Also to Deepen, practice...

STRETCHING TIGER VARIATION

The back bend is as deep as you desire. Kick into the hand and away from the buttocks, opening the shoulder, neck and chest.

Counter poses
- Cat–Cow
- Child's Pose
- Lying on belly with one cheek on the mat
- Downward Facing Dog
- Lord of the Fish
- Fish
- Bridge
- Upward Bow / Wheel
- Shoulder Stand or other arm balances

UPWARD PLANK POSE (PURVOTTANASANA)

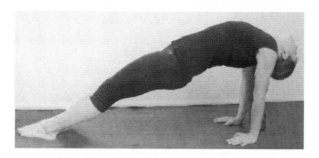

Getting into the Posture

1. From Staff pose, bend your knees so the soles of the feet are on mat and feet are a couple of feet in front of the pelvis.
2. Place the palms behind you on the ground, about shoulder-width apart with the fingers facing the hips.
3. With hands and feet grounded into the earth, allow the strength of the shoulders and legs to lift the pelvis upward, aligning the ankles under the knees (Stay here for Upward Table Top).
4. Without losing the height of the hips, slowly straighten out one leg at a time.
5. Gently lower your head to drop (in either variation) as much as your neck allows. If you have a healthy neck, your gaze may be entirely behind you, allowing the throat, chest and shoulders to open completely.

Modification

- Use blocks against the wall and/or on top of a non-slip surface, or mat under hands and/or feet.
- Use blocks/prop under the sacrum.
- Remain in Bridge until shoulders open and strength is gained.
- Use an exercise ball, pillow, ottoman, or similar prop to lay back on and allow the heart to open and lift.
- Do not lift the hips; focus instead on lifting the chest and collarbone. If neck allows, drop the head back, slowly opening the throat and neck as well.
- Practice Upward Table Top (Ardha Purvottanasana).

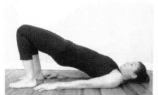
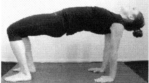

Remain in Bridge　　　　　　　　　　Upward Table Top

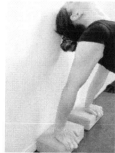
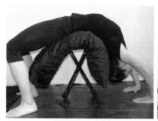
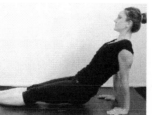

Blocks against wall　　Props to assist　　Hips stay down, focus on opening shoulders and chest

Deepen

- Press into the earth, lifting entire front body toward the sky; engage entire legs and buttocks. Continue to use the breath to lift and expand energetically through the collarbone and the heart center.
- May also use a block in between thighs to engage the inner thighs and hamstrings.
- Flow moving the hips with slow control up and down.

To further deepen...

EXTENDED BALANCING UPWARD TABLE TOP

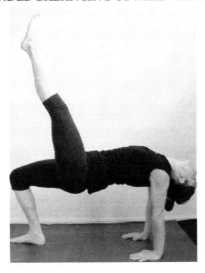

EXTENDED BALANCING PLANK

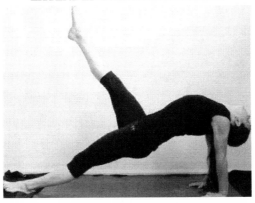

Also practice...

WILD THING (CAMATKARASANA)

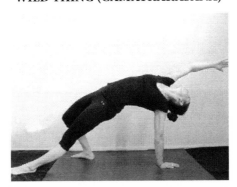

Getting into the Posture
1. From Upward Table Top, extend one leg out long.
2. Bring the other back foot behind you.
3. Pointing the front foot and pressing the sole of the foot into the earth, reach the top arm upward and backward reaching behind your head to elongate the entire front body.
4. Continue to open and stretch the entire front body and lift; engage the entire backside.

SCALE POSE (TOLASANA)

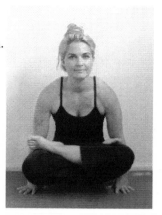

Inhale poise, stability and fortitude. Exhale weakness and fatigue. Feel the grounding, stable and balancing sensations of this posture. Realize just how truly strong you are in the Lord. Inhale HIS strength.

Getting into the Posture

1. From Simple Seated (or Half/Full Lotus), place hands on floor next to hips.
2. On an inhalation, using your core strength, bring the body off the earth.
3. Hold for up to one minute or add push-ups.

Modification

- Place a block under each palm.
- Practice Simple Seated, Half or Full Lotus Seated.

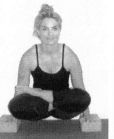 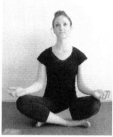 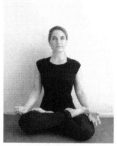

With blocks   Simple Seated   Seated Lotus

Deepen

- Practice leg variations and foot placements.

Also try...

ROOSTER POSE (KUKKUTASANA)

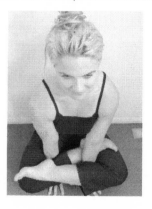

Getting into the Posture

1. From Simple Seated or Lotus, slip hands into the crease between the thighs and calves.
2. Lift legs and torso up.

Progress into…

ONE LEG OVER ARM BALANCE / ELEPHANT'S TRUNK (EKA HASTA BHUJASANA)

Allow your body and mind patience in this posture. Exhale disappointment and failure, while focusing on bringing in success and victory in all areas of your life.

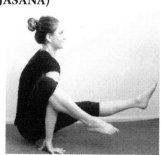

Getting into the Posture

1. Clasp one foot and place this leg as high up on the arm as possible. The knee will energetically "hug" the arm as you place both hands next to hips.
2. When you exhale, press palms into the earth as you lift the foundational leg and sitting bones off the earth.

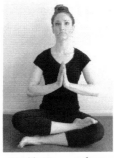

Modification

- Place a block under each palm.
- Practice Simple Seated or Double Pigeon Forward Fold; repeat on opposite side.
- Practice Scale.
- Continue to practice opening up the hip without raising the buttocks off the ground but getting the leg further up towards the shoulder.

With blocks

Double Pigeon to focus on hips

Deepen

- Practice leg variations and foot placements.
- Hold for one to two minutes before practicing the other side.
- Practice push-ups while in posture.

PLANK POSE (KUMBHAKASANA)

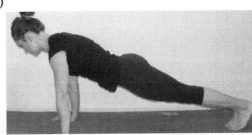

You may need to work up to this strong posture by practicing smaller lengths of time in the posture and taking breaks by coming down to your knees. Once you find your strength, continue to focus on bringing in endurance, stamina and determination. Your exhalations will help you become stronger and more fearless. Breathe in, embrace being fearless and strong.

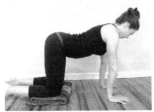

Modification

- Stand facing a wall. Place hands directly in front of you so wrists are straight out from shoulders; use the wall until enough strength is built up to come down to full posture on the ground.
- Place knees on floor, or use blanket under knees if extra padding is needed.
- Place bolster or similar prop under the sternum to gently assist in supporting torso.
- Practice Table Top.
- Practice Downward Facing Dog or Dolphin.
- Place a rolled-up towel under palms to alleviate wrist pain.

Practice Table Top

Deepen

- Lift one foot at a time and hold 30 seconds or more (Three-Legged Dog).
- Bring knee to meet nose, or elbow for a power move to sculpt and tone.
- Practice on forearms (Forearm Plank).
- Practice One Legged Arm Balance, knee touches the elbow and also engages inward toward the torso, back leg lifts off earth.

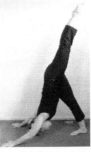

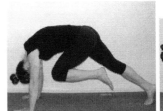

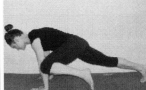

Knee to nose

Knee to elbow

Flow with 3 Legged Dog

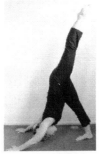

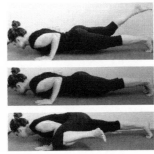

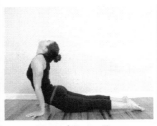

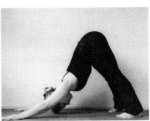

Flow with 3 Legged Dog

Low Plank

Upward Facing Dog (may also do Cobra)

Downward Facing Dog

172

SIDE PLANK / SIDE ARM BALANCE / LATERAL INCLINED PLANK (VASISTHASANA)

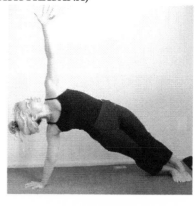

Progressing from Plank, roll to one side stacking the feet for Side Plank. Inhale a brand new mind set as your exhalations send out your old way of thinking. Feel your strength and stability as you let go of weakness and instabilities. Through Him, you are strong!

Modification

- Press the soles of the feet to a wall or a block against the wall; always stay buoyant in the hips.
- Bottom leg places the knee on the floor; foot faces behind you, using the core to lift, perhaps lifting the top leg up.
- Lean on the seat of a chair or similar prop.
- Balance on the lower forearm instead of hand.

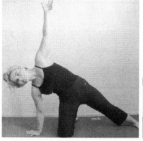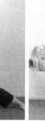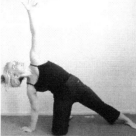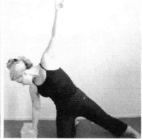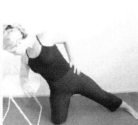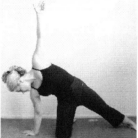

Knee stays on earth, gaze is down, forward or up	Knee on floor	Gaze down, use blocks	Seat of a chair	Face downward

Deepen

- Lift top leg up.
- Reach for the top leg's foot. (Breathe!)
- Reach top arm's bicep beyond the ear, lengthening throughout the entire side body.
- Top leg and arm reaches behind you, pressing the top of the foot so the heel and buttocks connect one day.
- Top leg comes into a Half Lotus position as the top hand reaches behind for a bind reaching for the Half Lotus foot.
- For these variations, you may also place the bottom knee on the floor; foot faces behind you and/or the forearm rests instead of hand.

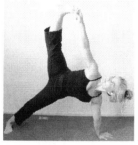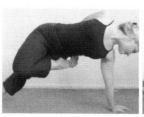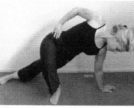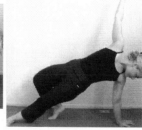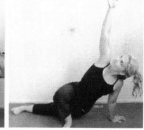

Lift top leg up   Bind reaching for the Half Lotus foot   Add vinyasa flow by "dipping" the hip down with control, leg can be in front or back

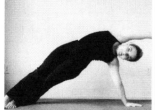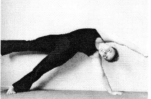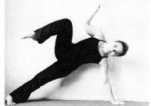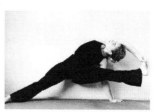

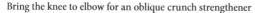

Bring the knee to elbow for an oblique crunch strengthener   Yet another variation and arm balance

Also practice…

FOUR-LIMBED STICK POSE / LOW PLANK (CHATURANGA DANDASANA)

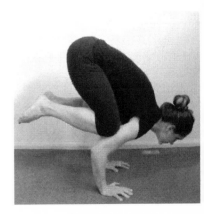

Inhalations focus on stamina and fortitude. As you exhale, send out weakness, "can't," instability and any imbalances.

Getting into the Posture
1. From High Plank, allow the elbows to hug the rib cage as you slowly lower down to hover above the earth.
2. Bring the navel in and upward; the entire front, back and side bodies are strong and engaged.
3. Energetically press through the heels.
4. Energetically lift the hamstrings upward.

Modification
- Stand facing a wall. Place hands directly in front of you so wrists are straight out from shoulders. Use the wall until you build up enough strength to come down to full posture on the ground.
- Place knees on floor, or use blanket under knees if you need extra padding.
- Place bolster or similar prop under the sternum to gently assist in supporting torso.
- Place rolled-up towel under palms to alleviate wrist pain.

Deepen
- Lift one foot at a time.
- Roll onto the balls of your feet, shifting your torso forward as hands come in closer to body, increasing front body stretch.
- Practice vinyasa by flowing into variations with Three-Legged Dog, Son Salutations, Abdominal and Oblique crunches to center and side.
- Bring leg to the outside of the elbow; engage the arm with the knee. Let your heart come toward the earth as you bend the elbows, perhaps coming into One-Legged Arm Balance (Eka Pada Koundinyasana II).

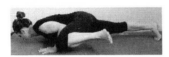
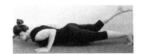
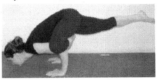

Knee to elbow   Lift leg and hold   One-Legged arm balance

CRANE / CROW (BAKASANA)

Getting into the Posture
1. From Mountain Pose, bring feet about hip-width apart.
2. Bend the knees deeply to come into a deep squat; place hands shoulder-width apart and come onto the balls of the feet. Come to the tops of the toes as much as you can.
3. Bring the knees into the armpits as you create a "shelf" with the triceps.
4. Spread all ten fingers apart wide and gently bend the elbows.
5. Come higher to the tops of the toes, lifting them completely off the earth someday.

Modification
- Use a block or similar prop to firm the toes on, to assist with support.
- Stay in low squat for Crow Prep.
- Place a block to rest the forehead on.
- Practice Baby Crow (Karandavasana) by coming onto the forearms.

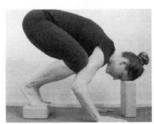
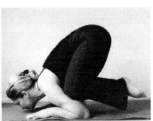

Use blocks under feet and forehead   Baby Crow

Deepen

- "Tuck" yourself in tighter; place the big toes to gently touch.
- From Crow, jump back into Yoga Push-Up (Chataranga Dandasana).
- Continue to spread all ten fingers out for a solid foundation, and deeply engage the inner groin into the pelvis to create "lift" and strength.
- Practice Half Crow, use your core strength to extend and lift one leg off the arm. Practice with bent arms and move into straightening the arms someday, or continue extending both legs upward for Handstand.

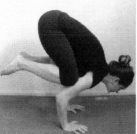 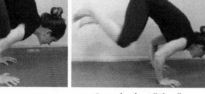 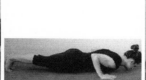 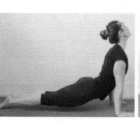 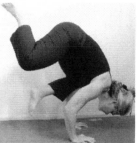

| Crow | Jump back to "Flow" | Low Plank | Deeply engage groins into the pelvis to create "lift" | Half Crow |

SIDE CROW (PARSVA BAKASANA)

Getting into the Posture

1. From Revolved Chair, squat deeply so heels and buttocks are touching, or close to touching.
2. Place the hands on the outside of thighs, while feet and knees continue to face forward.
3. May use a block to elevate the feet.
4. Gently bend the elbows, creating a "shelf" with both triceps for the outer thigh.
5. Come to the tops of the toes as much as possible, someday lifting them off the earth.

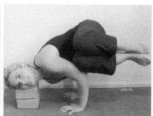

Modifications

- Practice Side Crow Prep.
- Practice with as many props as necessary.

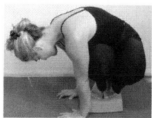 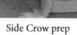

| Side Crow prep | Side Crow modified |

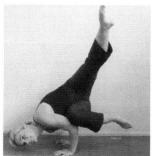 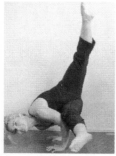

Deepen

- Extend one or both legs.
- Hold for 2 minutes.

One leg extends   Both legs extended

PEACOCK (MAYURASANA)

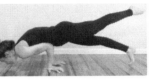

Getting into the Posture

1. From Table Top, turn the fingertips toward the feet, trying to keep both palms on the earth. Pinky fingers may touch, or you can separate hands.
2. Create a "shelf" with the elbows as your torso lowers down.
3. Allow the elbows to root upward into the belly.
4. Using the core, extend and lift the legs out. You may practice one leg at a time as well.
5. Gaze is on the earth. Elbows, forearms and palms remain connected to the ground.
6. Energetically engage the elbows toward one another. Breath is relaxed.

Modification

- Keep both feet on ground.
- Practice Legs up the Wall.
- Use a wall for legs or feet; practice releasing one foot at a time, or both feet stay on ground (Halfway version or Dolphin on the forearms) until you're confident to release both.
- Practice Half Shoulder Stand or Plow.
- Place blocks or bolster between hands and rest the top of the head on prop, as well as one or both feet on props.
- Separate the hands.

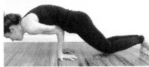
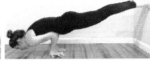

Keep both feet on ground   Place feet on wall   Only one leg lifts

Deepen

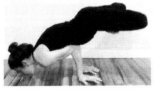

- Practice leg variations, such as Lotus or Half Lotus.

Peacock with Lotus legs

FIREFLY (TITTIBHASANA)

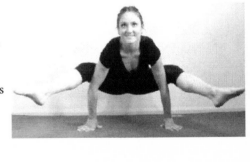

Getting into the Posture

1. From Mountain Pose, step your feet hip-width, or slightly wider than hip-width apart.
2. Forward fold, deeply tucking your shoulders behind the knees.
3. Frame the heels with the index finger and thumb while lowering into a deep squat.
4. Shift your weight onto the hands as you lift the legs off the earth, straightening them as much as possible.

Modification

- Place a block under each palm.
- Forward Fold with hands between legs and "cupping" heels in-between the thumbs and index fingers. Continue to engage in this position.
- Sit on floor; raise heels on blocks as you press hands into the earth between your legs.
- Stand on blocks and fold down, feeling the sensations of this posture until you trust yourself enough to lift the toes off the earth or blocks.

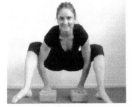
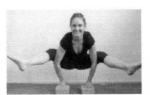
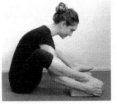
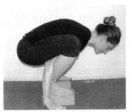

Blocks under palms, legs stay bent   Blocks with extended legs   Seated hip opener   Firefly prep with blocks

ARM BALANCING POSTURES

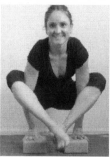

Firefly Variation

Deepen

- Practice leg variations and foot placements.
- One example: Bring tailbone to hover above the earth, as legs are straight and pointing towards the sky (as shown).
- Move from Firefly, into Crow, into Chaturanga Dandasana or Son Salutation.
- Hold posture until fatigued.

To further deepen the posture, practice…

ARM PRESSING POSE (BHUJAPIDASANA)

Getting into the Posture

1. Legs are placed as high on the arms as possible. Much like Firefly, with all the same great benefits.
2. Legs continue to engage the arms while you lock your feet together.
3. Perhaps try push-ups here.
4. A gradual shifting of the center of your gravity will help you stay lifted and buoyant.

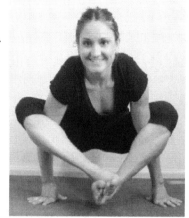

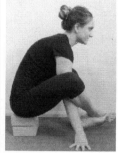

Modifications with blocks

Deepen

- Practice Shoulder Pressing Pose to Firefly, to Crow; jump back into Vinyasa Flow.

But He said to me, "My grace is sufficient for you, for My power is made perfect in weakness."
Therefore, I will boast all the more gladly about my weaknesses, so that Christ's power may rest on me. 2 Corinthians: 12:9

ELBOW BALANCE / FOREARM STAND / FEATHERED PEACOCK (PINCHA MAYURASANA)

In your deepest expression of this posture, let go of any vanity or pride. Like a peacock, think about the fact that you are distinguished and set apart. Continue to breathe in humility. Embrace your creativity and artistic side as you exhale any lethargy or self-doubt. Embrace your strong, beautiful self without letting pride or boasting creep in. You are sanctified, set apart for holy purposes.

Getting into the Posture

1. Begin in Dolphin pose; shoulder blades are engaged down toward the tailbone and focus on "hugging" the front ribs to the torso, all ten fingers spread apart.
2. Begin to walk your feet up towards the chest, while shifting the weight forward and allowing the forearms to "settle in" and bear the weight.
3. When you can no longer walk the feet in any further, bring both feet upward, or bending one knee at a time, extend one leg at a time. If you bring one knee/foot up at a time, be careful not to shift your weight extremely onto one side of the neck. Bringing both feet up at once will increase your strength for the full expression of Feathered Peacock. Keep in mind this is also called Forearm Balance; your forearms are the foundation of the posture.
4. Lengthen through the legs, engaging them inward as if you were standing in Mountain Pose. You want to be vertical as if you were standing upright; back is straight, breathe and lengthen.
5. Let the energy "sink down," allow your breath to be steady.

Continued on page 178.

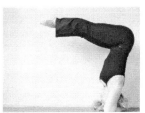

Inverted Staff, may place feet on
the wall

Modification

- Practice Legs up the Wall, Downward Facing Dog, Plow or Inverted Staff (with a wall in each if needed).
- Use a chair, similar prop or a large exercise ball to drape yourself over to feel the sensation of being upside down.
- Hang your head off the edge of your bed, perhaps move to hanging the torso off the edge.
- Practice Tripod Headstand (with or without the wall).
- Stay in Dolphin, focus on hugging the front ribs into the torso and engaging the core. Practice jumping heels to buttocks with control, then progress to extending one leg at a time upward.

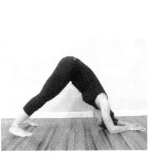 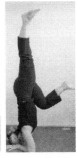 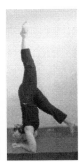 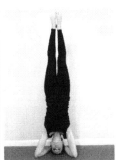

Dolphin, focus on
core engagement

One leg at a time

Tripod Headstand

Deepen

- Continue to allow your energy to sink down into the forearms; energetically engage the elbows inward toward one another as you press them into the earth.
- Practice various leg positions, Half or Full Lotus, widen legs, bend legs forward and backward, etc.
- Hold for 2 minutes or longer (only for experienced practitioners).
- Come into Scorpion Legs, feet come backward towards or beyond the head, then come into Wheel, stand up in Mountain from Wheel to complete an invigorating sequence.

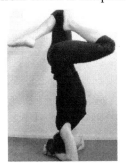 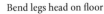 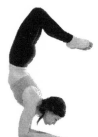 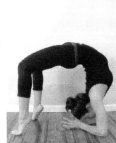 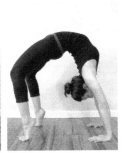 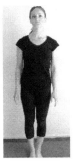

Bend legs head on floor   1. Scorpion   2. Wheel Variation   3. Wheel   4. Mountain

To further progress from Elbow Balancing Posture, practice…

SCORPION POSE (VRSCHIKASANA)

Getting into the Posture

1. From Feathered Peacock, slide the scapulae together on the back. This will lower the rib cage and increase mobility in the thoracic spine.
2. As you lift your head, your weight will shift in balance.
3. Allow your energy and breath to settle before bending the knees, bringing the feet closer to the head, or perhaps to touch the head.

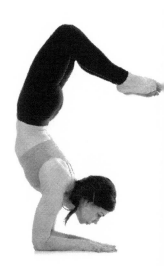

EIGHT ANGLE POSE (ASTAVAKRASANA)

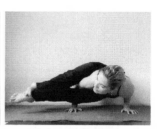

Getting into the Posture

1. Start with cradling one knee into the crease of the elbow, bringing the inside of the leg into the torso, perhaps to touch. Keep the spine tall. Hold this posture for several breaths, opening up the hips, chest and shoulders. As you engage the leg into your heart center with every breath, clasp the wrists or fingers tightly around the front of the leg to warm up fingers, hands and wrists.

2. Tuck your shoulder, as much as possible, under the cradled leg's knee; come back to a lengthened spine and torso.

3. Place each hand on the ground (or on blocks) next to your hips.

4. Bring the foot that is still on the earth up to lock ankles and feet together in front of torso. This lock is your bind; it will secure your legs so that you can remain in the posture without your legs and feet separating. Keep them locked tightly.

5. On an inhalation, simultaneously lift the tailbone off the earth.

6. On an exhalation, bend the elbows as you lower the torso down toward the earth and extend the legs at to the side. Final expression is to look at the feet.

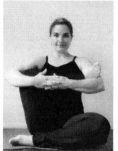
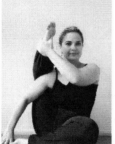
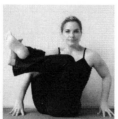
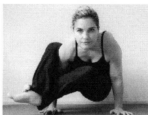

| 1. Leg Cradle | 2. Tuck shoulder | 3. Lock ankles, lift legs | 4. Inhale lift tailbone | 5. Exhale extend legs outward |

Modification

- Stay in Cradle Pose (placing one foot inside the opposite elbow crease and hugging in towards the torso).
- Use a block or similar prop on outside hip and leg for support, and/or under each palm.

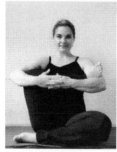
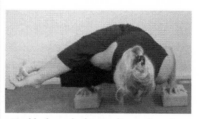

Use blocks under hips and/or under palms

Leg cradle

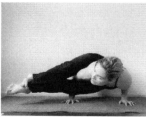

Practice push ups or hold 2 minutes

This is a challenging posture and the quintessential pose of the arm balance asana family. Once you obtain this posture, simply make sure your breath is steady and mind is calm. *Feel* how amazingly strong Christ created you to be!

Deepen

- Perform push-ups.
- Hold 1-2 minutes.

My help comes from the Lord, the maker of heaven and earth. Psalm 121:2

FLYING PIGEON / ONE LEGGED SAGE BALANCE 1/A (EKA PADA GALAVASANA)

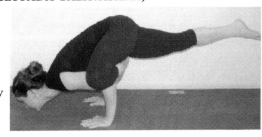

Getting into the Posture

1. From Tip Toe Pose (may also come from High Plank or Downward Facing Dog), place the palms on the ground in front of you, spreading all ten fingers.
2. On an exhalation, softly bend the elbows, creating a "shelf" with your tricep area.
3. Bring your heart towards the earth as you extend the back leg upward. Energetically lift the entire backside towards the sky. Breath is calm and steady.

Modification

- Use a block or similar prop under hands or head.
- Practice Planks, or focus on an arm balance that you have already done successfully.
- Practice Tip Toe or Side Crow.
- Practice Low Plank Knee to Elbow.

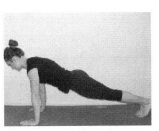
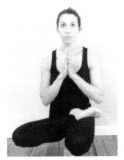
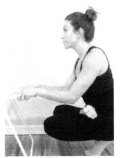
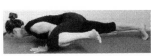

Low Plank knee to elbow

Practice High Plank or
Forearm Plank

Tip Toe modified

Tip Toe

Deepen

- Hold up to 2 minutes.
- Leg lifts with the back leg.
- Perform push-ups.

Once you obtain this posture, make sure your breath is steady and mind is calm. Feel how amazingly strong your body is.

To further progress, practice…

ONE LEGGED SAGE ARM BALANCE 2/B (EKA PADA KOUNDIYANASANA II)

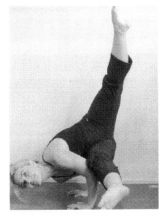

Getting into the Posture

1. From Flying Pigeon, extend the lower leg.
2. Lengthen both legs outward. Final expression of this posture is to look out instead of down or forward.

Inhale gratitude that the same resurrection power that rose Jesus from the grave resides in you!

These things I have spoken unto you, that in Me you might have peace.
In the world, you shall have tribulation: but be of good cheer; I have overcome the world. John 16:33

Prayer:
Thank you Lord that the weaker I am, the stronger You act on my behalf! I rest in knowing that You are my victory, protection and strength. All I ever have to do is "stand still." Lord, remind me when I am trying to do things in my own strength. I know this only leads to failure and frustration. Whisper to my soul, "Surrender, let Me handle it." I surrender my will and my way to You Father; have Your way in my heart today! With every breath Lord, may I always glorify, honor and praise You! In Jesus' name I pray, Amen!

A FINAL NOTE: OBTAINING WHOLENESS

Now that you have experienced the physical, mental, emotional and spiritual benefits of YogaFaith and intimacy with Christ, how will you continue to seek and obtain this new found wholeness?

Will you continue your daily appointment with God? Will you meditate on His promises throughout the day and begin to possess the promises? Will you continue your path to completeness, perhaps leading your family and others to experience the same? Who can you share your new discoveries with and bring into your new world?

I want to challenge you to continue to apply the knowledge you have acquired during our time together and keep at it. What other activity can you do where you get rest, meditation, movement, whole worship and complete surrender, all in one activity such as YogaFaith? The bonus is weight loss, a balanced life, calmness, consistent moods, anti-aging (hello inversions), and most importantly, hearing the voice of God.

I challenge you to resist the urge to "do," to gather, produce, work and 'accomplish' every day of the week. This challenge is to find rest. Find His perfect Sabbath rest at least one day of the week; make it a day where you cease, stop and withdraw. Continue to exchange activities that do not move you toward the dreams God has placed in your heart (even if they are good activities) for tasks that align with His Word and your destiny.

EXERCISE:
Write ten exchanges that you commit to replacing over the next 90 days.

Example: I commit to exchange the snooze time to meditating with God, the first fruit of my morning, at least 5 minutes every day. [Side Note: Choose a time that works best for you; it doesn't have to be the exact time each day, just make it happen. Schedule it as an appointment in your planner or set an alarm on your phone. Don't miss this urgent, daily and vital appointment.]

1._____

2._____

3._____

4._____

5._____

6._____

7._____

8._____

9._____

10._____

If you want to continue the physical, mental, emotional, spiritual and relational benefits that the practice of YogaFaith brings, you should include the action item of practicing one to five postures a day, then have fun and create your own personal sequencing as your own act of worship to the Lord. Take another action of creating play lists and themes as your worship time with God. It is amazing that when you need rest, for example, you have songs that focus on rest and being still while you practice seated or restorative postures. If you're weary, have a playlist ready to go at any given moment on strength, renewal, and a powerful, flowing sequence that you can access at any time. God is not boring, so have fun as you create time with Him.

You can take these actions a step further and include your family and friends. Have a YogaFaith class on the deck while the sun sets, or come together once a month for a bible study and class. You can practice YogaFaith on Friday nights with your family as a time to have fun, worship and enjoy one another. I like to share scriptures, dig in the Word and discuss this with whomever is present. Sometimes it might just be you and your spouse. What an awesome time together, using each other in postures and pursuing God together. Now you have created intimacy in your family and set an example of taking time for the Lord. This habit can be passed to other generations, who will become healthy, whole and united as family.

A FINAL NOTE

The enemy loves to work in our families; if he can divide families, then he will win. We can stop this and declare our families have been paid for with the blood of Jesus. What if we cooked meatloaf every night for our families? Of course, they'd become bored. I often think God probably tires of my "same old" prayer. I believe He appreciates various forms of praise, worship and prayers. Have fun together worshiping the Lord and making Him the center of your home. Will you commit to making Jesus the center of your family, and not just a Sunday morning God?

In our time together, you have learned to be still, to listen and be sensitive to the Holy Spirit. You have learned about obtaining balance in our often-hectic daily lives. You have experienced the biblical and vital practice of meditation and chanting, or melodic praise. You have learned how to worship with your entire being, the freedom of moving and flowing with the Lord in His perfect, amazing love and grace. You have experienced transformation and the many benefits of stretching your physical body, as well as trusting Him and stretching your faith and spirit. When you continue to seek Him wholeheartedly, you will find Him. You will continue to preserve success in all these areas and set an example for others in your family and community, ultimately leading them to transformation, and most importantly, to the Heart of God.

Now that you've completed this book, please connect with me, as our journey together has just begun. I love to meet my eternal family before we get to Heaven and would also love to hear what you enjoyed or perhaps didn't enjoy so much. Arm balances are off limits, you'll enjoy them someday I promise, maybe in Heaven! Your feedback will help me improve the next edition of *Stretching Your Faith*.

I want to link arms with you and walk through the mountaintops as well as the valleys with you. Tell me where you are in your journey, with life, family, God or no God, your adversities and obstacles. Tell me how I can help you. Perhaps we can connect by phone, email, or you can book me to travel to your location to speak for your organization or lead a YogaFaith class or training.

As a way for us to stay connected, I invite you to "Like" YOGAFAITH on Facebook, or my personal page MichelleAnnThielen. You may also email me directly at michelle@yogafaith.org, include your name and time zone to connect via phone or Skype. If geography allows, I'd love to meet you personally.

I wish you all the success in the world! The most important thing is that you know God has greatness in store for you. He wants you to be successful! He needs you to know that you were created for a specific purpose and destiny, and nothing you have done or could ever do will detour you from His predestined plan for your life. If it were just you on earth, nothing would have changed at the cross. God would have sent His one and only begotten Son to die for you so you can live a life of freedom and abundance. Isn't this the most phenomenal news ever? Don't let what Christ paid such a high price for be squandered for one more day.

I will pray for your peace, balance, and freedom in Christ. I pray that through the Christ-centered practice of YogaFaith, you will continue to hear His voice on and off a yoga mat. God's plan for your life works best when you hear from Him. I am excited about your future! I expect all the goodness of Christ to manifest in your life starting right now! I look forward to hearing about it face to face in the future.

With all my heart and soul, your friend,

Michelle Thielen

THE RESTORATION OF MODERN DAY SLAVES: THE HEART OF YOGAFAITH'S MINISTRY

Human trafficking is the illegal trade of human beings, mainly for the purposes of forced labor and sex trafficking. As the world's fastest growing criminal industry, it affects every nation across the globe. Every 30 seconds, someone becomes a victim of modern-day slavery. There are more slaves in the world today than at any other point in human history, with an estimated 27 million in bondage across the globe. Men, women, and children are being exploited for manual and sexual labor against their will (Source: A21, 2015).

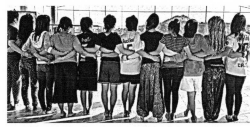
Picture of YogaFaith & traffick survivors at Destiny Rescue,
ChaingRai, Thailand 2014

I first learned of human trafficking in 2008 while watching a Joyce Meyer session. It was the first time that I heard of girls, as young as 5 years old, servicing up to 20 men on a daily basis. My stomach churned and I ended up on my living room floor weeping with a broken heart for these souls that I didn't know personally, but I knew each one had a name. I imagined myself at five years old, what life was like through the innocence of my childhood. Dancing and dolls, playing with my friends and climbing trees with my brothers. It's difficult to comprehend that such atrocity was happening and not just in third world countries, but in our own backyards in America. Through my tears I began to lift these precious souls up to the Lord. I vowed to Him, and myself, that for the rest of my life I would do all that I personally could to combat the evils of human trafficking.

We cannot do anything about anything if we do not know about it. But once we know, we can implement change. You see, God's people are destroyed for their lack of knowledge (See Hosea 4:6), and in these perilous times we cannot afford to be ignorant. In 2008 I joined forces with an organization out of Vancouver, WA: Shared Hope International. I became an Ambassador of Hope helping to raise awareness and share this epidemic with the world. Shared Hope International was established by Washington State Congresswoman Linda Smith, founded in 1998. Shared Hope International strives to prevent the conditions that foster sex trafficking, restore victims of sex slavery, and bring justice to vulnerable women and children. They are a committed community restoring survivors to lives of purpose and value, one life at a time.

SINCE 2006 TO PRESENT TIME, ANNUALLY, SLAVE OWNERS HAVE MADE MORE MONEY THAN GOOGLE, STARBUCKS AND NIKE COMBINED.

In 2013, friends, family and partners of YogaFaith allowed me the privilege to travel to Bulgaria and Greece with the A21 Campaign. Founded by Christine Caine in 2007, A21 exists to abolish injustice in the 21st century through a comprehensive system; achieving preventative measures to help potential victims evade trafficking, victim protection through shelters and aftercare programs, prosecution of violators, and strategic partnerships. During my time in Bulgaria and Greece, we were able to spread awareness and have a hands-on approach to helping the survivors throughout these parts of the world.

In 2014, YogaFaith students and our local community made it possible to travel to Cambodia and Thailand to share YogaFaith with local organizations such as Destiny Rescue and others in Asia. Our team was able to share Christ and the healing power of YogaFaith with those that have survived human trafficking. We were able to spend a great amount of time with these young girls and boys. We witnessed true transformation that could have only been done through God's love, and their surrendered hearts. YogaFaith helped them to release their trauma and allow the Lord to take their ashes and turn them into something so beautiful. It was a profound experience for them as well as myself. I left Asia changed.

In 2015 our class donations have reached our local community in the Pacific Northwest, meeting needs for survivors and shelters where they live when transitioning from off the streets. Profits from *every product* in the YogaFaith.org store go towards the fight against human trafficking. We are involved in every aspect of anti-trafficking: Raising awareness, changing and implementing laws, as well as rescuing, clothing, feeding, housing and educating victims.

YogaFaith is a nonprofit that relies on assistance from those who believe in our mission and vision of restoring these survivors' lives. We cannot share the message of grace, hope and restoration without your help. YogaFaith is a powerful vehicle to whole transformation and true healing. We thank you for helping this ministry and I, personally thank you that we can continue this vital work around the world.

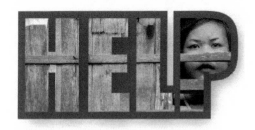

WHAT YOU CAN DO

- Get the facts, share the facts.
- Partner with your local church or organization to host raising awareness nights or start a street outreach.
- Organize a group to pray prayer circles around local trafficking sites, never alone.
- Volunteer at a local traffick organization.
- Donate to YogaFaith or anyone involved in helping victims.
- Purchase any item at YogaFaith.org
- Pray for victims, survivors, organizations, law enforcement and anyone involved in this epidemic. Those on the front lines face immense challenges everyday. Often law enforcement is involved in protecting brothels and the victims, never forget the power of prayer!
- Host an informative night at your house with friends and family.
- Host a YogaFaith class or a healthy living workshop in your community to raise awareness or financial aid for a local trafficking shelter or a YogaFaith mission trip.
- Be a part of YogaFaith's next mission trip.

We may not be able to do much, but each of us can do something.

Thank you for learning and "stretching your faith" beyond borders to help others. We are a blessed people and our blessings are no good unless we are doing something with them. So now that you know, what will you do to help? I encourage you to get outside of your world and walk in the shoes of those less fortunate. I promise you there is a blessing on the other side of serving others and extending yourself.

Learn more at Yogafaith.org.

"When you learn, teach, when you get, give." **Maya Angelou**

YOGAFAITH TRAINING PROGRAM

If you want to deepen your walk with God and increase your personal yoga practice, then become an internationally accredited yoga instructor through YogaFaith. If you're ready to start living up to your maximum capacity, YogaFaith's Training Program is the next step toward your destiny. There is no better time than now to start clearing out the clutter of the past and create space for new things from God. Are you ready for the B.I.G., the Blessings In God?

Not only can you learn to be a sought-after yoga trainer, you can gain vital tools necessary to change your world. Develop the unique gifts and talents God placed within you. Use the confidence God gave you to implement them. You are the one that God has chosen. He has promised that you are the one to set captives free, heal the brokenhearted and bring good news wherever you go (See Isaiah 61).

You are invited to enter into a true and lasting transformation with the Lord. His Spirit beckons your spirit to draw nearer to His heart and to stand out from the rest, sanctified and holy for a time such as this.

Allow Michelle Thielen, founder of the internationally recognized ministry of YogaFaith, author of *Stretching Your Faith*, to guide you through the process of becoming whole in your mind, body, spirit and soul. Over the course of more than 20 years, Michelle has trained thousands of students and instructors with studies and practice that focus on Christ and His word. There is no other program like YogaFaith. Allow Michelle to encourage, ignite and spark the dreams God has placed inside you to implement change within you and your world.

During your infinite journey with the YogaFaith Program, you will have unlimited access, an easy-to-follow road map and blueprint to the YogaFaith Program, Michelle, and The YogaFaith Family. YogaFaith takes any guesswork out and simplifies training like no other program. This program allows you to go at your own pace and study from the comfort of your home, with an optional, hands-on training. We are an eternal family, linked together as many imperfect people serving a perfect God. We want to "do life" with you... forever!

For more information, please visit Michelle online. Any questions regarding a YogaFaith Training, you can send directly to teachertraining@yogafaith.org.

www.YogaFaith.org · www.StretchingYourFaith.com · www.MichelleThielen.com

YOGAFAITH AMBASSADOR CIRCLE

Michelle Thielen offers an inclusive membership for her students, readers, trainers, and audiences who wish to create their own destinies in alignment with what God predestined for them. If you want to live with purpose, lead others to Christ, enjoy the "sweet spot" that He has for you, travel to share the gospel, as well as train up other YogaFaith trainers throughout the world, this circle is for you. Join other YogaFaith Ambassadors (YF-A) in sharing the message of grace, hope and the love of Christ around the world.

YogaFaith Ambassador Circle Benefits:
1. Living a life on purpose, with boldness and God-confidence.
2. Access to all training materials.
3. Access to all virtual studies.
4. Invitation to travel abroad.
5. Become a YogaFaith Master Trainer (R-YFMT), a trainer to the trainers.
6. Host Teacher Trainings (US and Abroad).
7. Be a Lead Trainer at YogaFaith's main Teacher Trainings.
8. Coordinate YogaFaith classes, events, workshops and retreats.
9. Travel to help in the rescue and restoration of human traffick survivors.
10. An integral role of an eternal family.

YogaFaith Ambassador Circle is a lifetime membership with no expiration date. When you become a YogaFaith Ambassador, you'll learn the sky is the limit and beyond...*way beyond!*

For more information visit YogaFaith.org/Ambassadors

ABOUT THE AUTHOR

MICHELLE THIELEN is an activist, author, professional speaker, business and life coach, and the founder of YogaFaith, a nonprofit ministry and internationally accredited Christian yoga school. She has trained thousands of students and instructors from around the world through classes, workshops, retreats and Yoga Alliance teacher trainings. She enjoys sharing the gift of yoga globally as a Shared Hope Ambassador, presenter of Yoga Alliance workshops and international yoga festivals. She holds a certification with The American Council of Exercise and is an International Registered Master Yoga Trainer with over 20,000 teaching hours.

Originally from Portland, Oregon, Michelle has always loved movement. At the age of five, she began with ballet slippers, which evolved into every kind of dance form. Eventually, she became a professional dancer and choreographer in numerous venues, including professional athletic teams such as the NBA and WNBA. She originally discovered yoga through dance, as she implemented its methods primarily for injury prevention, but then fell in love with the numerous benefits of the practice.

It has been more than 20 years since Michelle first discovered yoga. Throughout her studies and practice of various styles, her love of yoga, its community, and thousands of transformational testimonies gave her a passion for sharing the gift with others. Before falling in love with yoga, she fell in love with design. With a degree in Architecture and Design, Michelle worked for almost 20 years in the granite industry, helping others build their dreams. One day God said, "It is time to build the dreams I gave *you*."

Michelle's mission is to share the wonderful benefits of yoga and the healing power of Jesus Christ to a lost and hurting world. She believes it begins from within. If each one of us receives healing and wholeness we can then empower and ignite others to receive the same, creating a wildfire of revival throughout the globe.

For several years, Michelle has been an active ambassador and advocate with Shared Hope International, an organization that is changing laws and battling the root issues of human trafficking. She has also traveled with the A21 Campaign, an organization founded by Australian pastor Christine Caine, to help in the rescue efforts of today's slaves. Michelle's life mission is to abolish modern-day slavery, human trafficking and actualize justice in her generation. She offers donation-based classes so all people can enjoy yoga and community. Her prayer is that people will connect to Christ - on or off a yoga mat. All class donations go directly to international rescue and restoration efforts. Students, friends, and partners have sent the ministry of YogaFaith to many third world countries over the years to teach YogaFaith to young children. Michelle has seen the healing power of Jesus work in their lives. She knows they can be saved and restored. She looks forward to sharing yoga and Jesus, the hope for all humanity, to bring about true and lasting transformation in the lives of thousands more survivors, but also in your life.

In 2004, Michelle was deeply depressed and would not be here today without the redemptive power of Christ. She is grateful that God, and her mother, saved her from taking her own life. She knows now that she would have killed the wrong girl. "One day I woke up and decided to choose life, and I have never looked back," she says. She enjoys sharing her hope in God with others who are battling despair, discouragement and depression. There is hope! It is not always easy but it is always worth it!

God has blessed Michelle with the desires of her heart, including her soulmate and best friend, Derek Thielen. She and Derek live in the Seattle area with three, four-legged children; two dogs, Barkley Bear and Molly Girl, and a kitty named Steeler. In her free time she enjoys acting, modeling, dancing, traveling, reading and spa days.

GENTLE CLASS

YogaFaith Instructional Video Class Outlines, a companion to *Stretching Your Faith* book. To enjoy the 90 minute, 3 class instructional, go to YogaFaith.org/GetStretched enter password: SonWorshipper

3 ways to gently warm up:

1) GOOD MORNING GOD: (A great way to start your day in prayer but good anytime.)

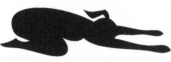

Inhale- High Mountain (Raise arms in Mountain) Hands through to heart center as you
Exhale- Forward Fold
Inhale- Bend knees (squat) as you sweep the earth with the back of your hands, rising up to
Exhale- High Mountain into
Inhale/Exhale- Standing Back bend, arms can be raised or on the small of your back
Repeat as much as desired.

Note: As your body warms up, your Forward Fold and squat should become deeper as well as your back bend.

2) GOOD AFTERNOON LORD: (Mid day stop and praise the Lord. May use anytime of the day.)

Inhale/Exhale- Child's Pose (Place blanket under knees if needed.)
Inhale- Table Top
Exhale- High to low push up (Hover above earth, use your muscles, we are trying to warm up the entire body here. Your exhalation takes you to the bottom of the push up, elbows hug rib cage.)
Inhale- Baby Cobra, Cobra or Extended Cobra (Toes point or connect to head.)
Exhale- Child's Pose

Note: This flow is a great alternative to Son Salutation A. Replacing the Downward Facing Dog with Table Top and the Upward Facing Dog with Cobra

3) GOOD EVENING FATHER: Thank you Lord for another day!

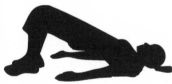

Lie in a Supine position, taking as many breaths as you need.
Inhale- Lift the hips to Bridge Pose
Exhale- Knees to Chest

Note: Flow in your own time and breath, there is no hurry here. Keep your entire spine rooted to the earth, when your knees come into the chest, do not pull the tailbone up. Knees to Chest pose is a powerful practice of your hands/arms pressing the toxins our of your internal organs. Stay present, not just going through the motions here. Bridge Pose, lift up and engage your entire backside.

SEATED
Neck Rolls- Drop right ear to shoulder, roll chin to chest, left ear to shoulder, keep a straight spine.
Wrist Stretches
Gentle twists, use as many props as needed
Staff Pose- Use props or deepen by Forward Folding or simply explore
Cow Face- Use Props or move the arms away from spine and forward fold to deepen
Seated Cat-Cow, may also use chair or practice from Table Top position

STANDING
Half Way Forward Fold, use chair or blocks if needed
Mountain with twists
Chair Pose

Warrior 1, Warrior II, Side Angle
Goddess to Garland

SUPINE
Knees to Chest, "Windshield Wiper" knees out for hip release. Right Leg into Chest, use strap if needed. Reclining Pigeon
Repeat on left side
Legs up the Wall
Resting Angel

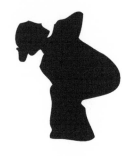

INTERMEDIATE CLASS

Warm Up
Mountain with leg/hip circles or warm up the hips another way
Mountain Twists
Mountain with Lateral Flexion (Side bends)
Son Salutation A
Chair with Twists and Side Crow Prep
Forward Fold with legs crossed, repeat other side

STANDING/BALANCE
Tree to Warrior III to Half Moon, repeat other side
Single Leg Swan, repeat other side

STRENGTH SEQUENCE

Mountain – Standing Forward Fold – Downward Facing Dog – 3 Legged Dog – Knee/Hip Circles – Wild Thing
3 Legged Dog – Low (or High) Lunge – Lateral Flexion – Finger/Eye Coordination Tuck – Grasshopper - Splits
Repeat on other side

Note: This is a great sequence to work the entire body. It will strengthen your hip joints mostly as well as improve your concentration, mental clarity, balance and muscle tone. Practice going as slow as you would like or stay in each posture as long as you would like.

Child's Pose – Cat-Cow – Table Top Arm Balance – Stretching Tiger, Repeat other side
Camel – Hero with Eagle Arms – Camel Reach Back

Child's Pose – Downward Facing Dog – walk through
Resting Angel

ADVANCED CLASS

Warm Up
Son Salutation B, 2 times (or more)

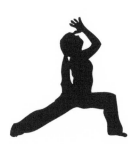

Chair – Chair Squats – Side Crow, Repeat on other side
Low or High Lunge – Warrior III – Upright Row (with or without hand weights) Repeat other side

Warrior I – Warrior II – Side Angle – Bicep Curls (with or without hand weights) Repeat other side
(In the video we only practice 5 repetitions once. As you gain strength I encourage you to do 8-12 repetitions up to 4 times per leg)
Standing Wide A Frame with lunges and optional weights
Revolved Standing Wide A Frame Forward Fold (Mild or deep twist)
(Head does not go below the heart if your heart rate is rapid)

Crow – Jump Back Chaturanga (Vinyasa flow) (Modify Crow with blocks and remain in this posture)
Crow – Tripod Headstand (Modify Crow to Standing Forward Fold, flow between these two postures)
8 Angle (Modify in Leg Cradle or Half Happy Baby until hips gain flexibility)

Legs up the Wall – Plow – Ear Pressure Pose – Revolved Plow on both sides

Legs up the Wall – Core Strengtheners: 30-60-90's – Resting Angel

Note: Practice additional core strengtheners by adding a "hold" and hover the feet above the earth for a 10 count, next, 30-60-90's, hold and scissor the legs slowly, repeat 30-60-90's and flutter the legs up and down slowly for a 10 count; on all of your 30-60-90's, make sure you pull the navel in toward the spine. Also, whenever you are at the 90 degree point with the legs, feet hovering about 3-4 inches from the earth, protect your spine by lifting the shoulder blades off the earth so that you gaze just beyond your toes.

I encourage you to explore these sequences further and create your own sequences that act as worship to your Creator. You will soon see how He enjoys you coming to Him with a new song, a new dance and a new way to pray.

Flow in His grace, forever and ever, Amen.

BOOK MICHELLE THIELEN TO SPEAK OR TEACH AT YOUR NEXT EVENT

Michelle Thielen has inspired thousands to reach their maximum potential and achieve true wholeness. Allow Michelle to help those at your event achieve lasting transformation from the inside out. Through Michelle's teachings, your audience, no matter how intimate or vast, will experience a peace, calm, healing, freedom and new found joy, along with a sense of purpose as they step forward into the destiny that God predestined for them.

Michelle is passionate about revival throughout the globe, encouraging and supporting each other and infusing joy into people. Her transparency and humor inspire audiences to stop living in fear, tear down walls, and heal the hurts that keep us from trusting and living the lives God meant us to lead. Michelle will encourage audiences to stop settling, dare them to use their strengths for change, justice and revival. When people find true wholeness within themselves, they can lead others to the same destination, sparking true change in the world.

Michelle will inspire, motivate, encourage and leave your audience truly transformed. To find out if Michelle is available to speak or teach YogaFaith at your next event, visit her online, or contact her directly by email.

www.YogaFaith.org · www.StretchingYourFaith.com · www.MichelleThielen.com
michelle@yogafaith.org

non YogaFaith inquiries please contact; Schedule@MichelleThielen.com